KETO CHAFFLE RECIPES COOKBOOK

The Ultimate Keto Food Guide for an Healthy, Lasting, & Tasty Weight Loss by Making Delicious, Quick & Easy Low Carb Keto Chaffles Recipes for Breakfast, Snacks & Dinner

JULIA WALKER

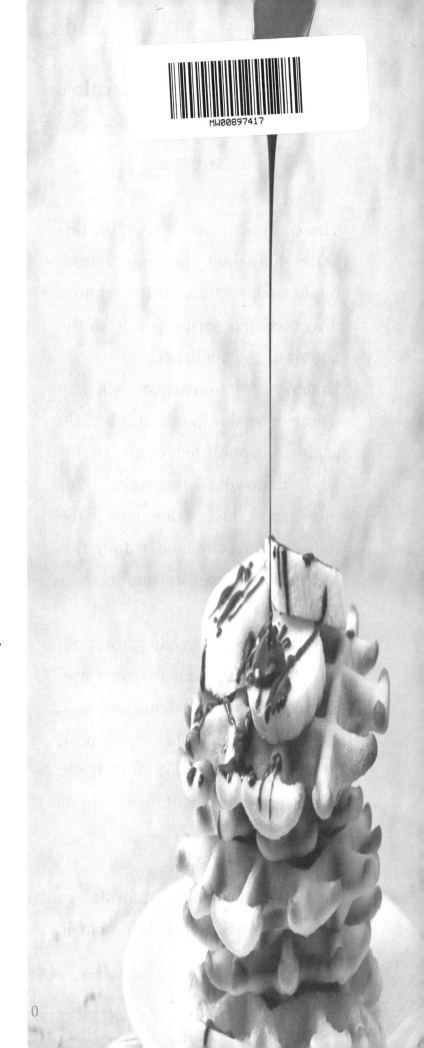

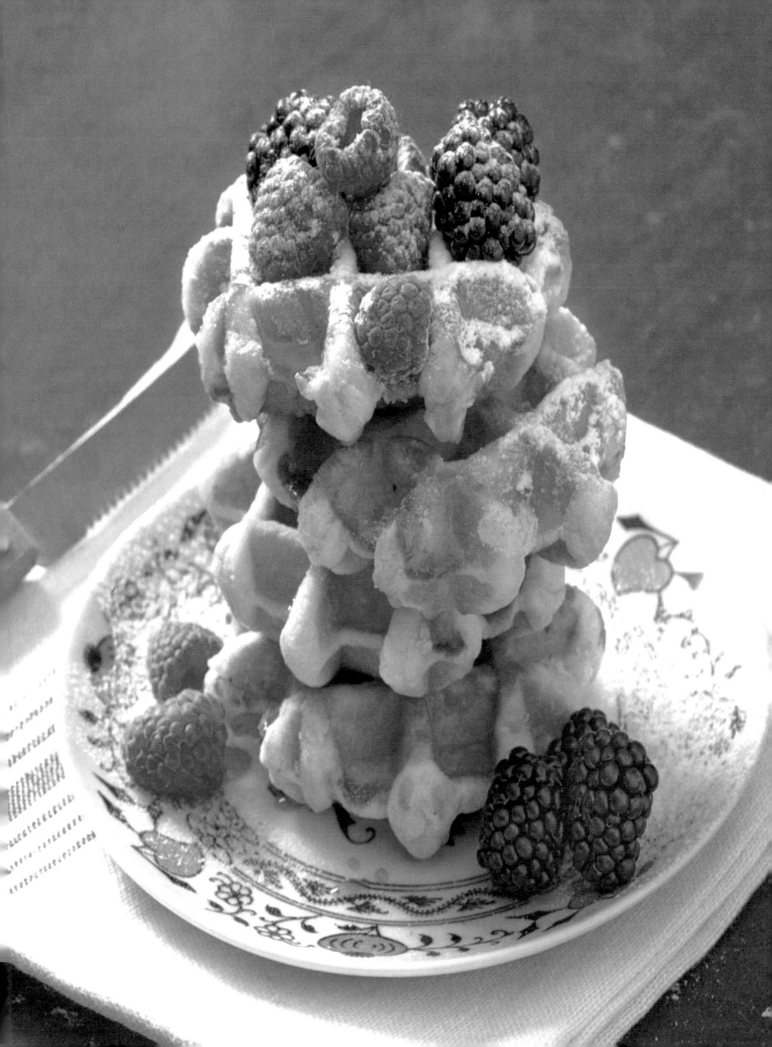

TABLE OF CONTENT

INTRODUCTION

Chaffles

You might have heard someone talking about eating chaffles, but you're not quite sure what it is. Chaffles are a tasty dish that combines two of the most delicious foods of all time—waffles and pancakes. If you love getting breakfast for dinner, then you'll love chaffles even more. These tasty treats are incredibly simple to make. The reason chaffles are so yummy is that waffles and pancakes both contain a lot of butter, which makes them rich in flavor. The syrup really brings out the flavor of both the waffles and the pancakes, just as it does when spread over maple waffles or on top of a stack of flapjacks. A chaffle requires no special equipment or ingredients to prepare. However, if you plan to make these tasty treats often, you may want to pick up some extra equipment. You'll need a waffle iron, which again can be found at any large grocery store for less than $30.

And finally, you'll want a giant pair of tongs. This tool has several different functions and will come in handy when you're making chaffles or even some other dishes—it's really a multipurpose kitchen utensil. The slotted side is meant for removing ice from drinks, while the other side is meant for chopping food. You can use the tongs to slide your chaffle off of the waffle iron or to flip it once it's folded. If you enjoy chaffles, you might want to try some of the other tasty, delicious dish recipes in this series. Crepes and waffles are a fantastic combination; in fact, many chefs like to combine these two foods to create common dishes. You can really experiment with all kinds of food combinations with crepes and waffles—they are an incredibly versatile food group!

Chaffles are really a great way to bring together two classic dishes into one fabulous meal. If you're a big fan of breakfast food, then you will absolutely love chaffles. All you need to prepare these tasty treats is a waffle iron and some pancake batter. Serve your chaffles with butter and syrup for a special breakfast treat – your family may even ask for seconds!

Why Chaffles Fit Well With a Keto Regime

If you're thinking about abandoning your diet because life is so full of carbs, stop worrying! All it takes is one glance at these awesome recipes to see all the yummy things you can eat on a keto diet. The truth is that if you're starting to get bored with eating chicken and veggies all the time, chaffles will probably be just what you need to start cooking healthier again.

Chaffles are a dish made from mashed

cauliflower and egg that tastes just like waffles. They're a fun keto breakfast alternative that will fill you up with good fat and protein. You can top them with whatever toppings you want; they're convenient and easy to make if you have cauliflower on hand.

These chaffles are crunchy on the outside and tender and sweet on the inside. They're delicious when served with a dollop of butter or a scoop of sugar-free ice cream. You can also pair them with fruit salad or fresh berries that are in season. Eating chaffles for breakfast will set your metabolism up for the day so that you can burn more calories than usual. This is possible because eating fat in the morning reduces your appetite later in the day and helps to manage blood sugar levels.

Chapter 1. Tips & Tricks to Make Amazing Chaffles

Gluten-free chaffles combine two of America's most popular foods, cheese, and waffles, and they appear everywhere on social media. They are the undisputed stars of many Pinterest forums and Instagram stories, and I've also found several recipe groups on Facebook with tens of thousands of members. Join one of them, and you'll be bombarded with an endless stream of gorgeous photos - and yes, most of them look truly delightful. While this concept is new to some of you, this overwhelming trend seems to have emerged across America. It occurs mainly in eaters on a limited diet. Really, who can blame them, the ketogenic diet lovers love to substitute for a low-carb, cheap, easy-to-make, completely grain-free bread.

Ready to jump to the bar? Basic chaffles only require a few daily ingredients—eggs and a handful of grated cheese with a little baking soda if desired to make it very light. Then you are limited only by your imagination and personal taste.

I personally prefer chaffle recipes that contain coconut or almond flour for a less moist taste (you can only use protein for the same effect). Extraordinary bread is even less spicy. Use mayonnaise as a binder, and it really tastes like soft white bread and pillow. Sweet spots are topped with cream cheese. Optional additions give special notes—for example, cocoa powder, vanilla, chocolate chips, and/or cinnamon as a dessert of turkey or meat slices, jalapeño slices, herbal spices, or more seasoned garlic spices. You can double up on the recipe below to make super tasty waffles (waffles are waffles, right?). But when you use it for sandwiches, the size of a mini waffle maker is perfect. Here are some tips for making perfect recipes: Preheat the waffle iron for a few minutes before using it and bring it to temperature.

Even if your waffle iron is brand new and has a whole Teflon coating, lightly spray the iron with cooking spray or melt the melted butter in all corners before adding the batter. Otherwise, the chaffles can jam.

Fill the hot iron with a light hand. The dough will come off after closing the lid, and if you mix it with the waffles, the dough will come out, leaving a terrible mess. Be patient. Resist the urge to open the waffle iron while you're cooking. If you're serving more than one serving, keep the grill hot and crisp in the oven at 200 degrees. Don't be afraid to be creative. Try different types of cheese, herbs, food supplements, and side dishes.

Do not check for soot or burning signs by opening the waffle iron too quickly! You want it to cook until ripe and crunchy. If nothing else, stretch the cooking side a little more than you think. You can certainly experiment with other cheeses that are good for keto—goat cheese and halloumi work well—but mozzarella is usually recommended because it's mild and not as high as other choices. If you want more protein and flavor, you can also add one slice of ham when mixing egg and cheese. Bacon can work, too (enough if you're on a strict keto diet). If you prefer sweet cubes, substitute the mozzarella cream. I like this tip! I can't imagine mozzarella on my cakes.

Sprinkle some extra cheese on the waffle iron before adding the egg and cheese mixture to get a warm, crispy crust.

It may be difficult to make it super crunchy on your plate because the steam from the stew softens them like all waves. It is best to eat or freeze them immediately, although I have found that a little almond flour helps the texture.

1. CHOCOLATE CHAFFLE

💜 **Servings:** 1

🧇 **Preparation Time**: 5 Minutes

⏰ **Cooking Time**: 5 Minutes

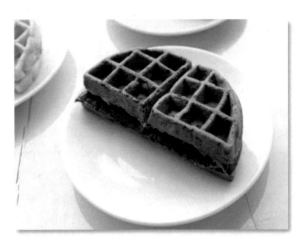

Ingredients:

- ✓ 2 tablespoons coconut flour
- ✓ 1 tablespoon cocoa powder
- ✓ 1 egg, whisked
- ✓ 1-ounce cream cheese, soft
- ✓ 1 teaspoon vanilla extract
- ✓ 1 tablespoon stevia

Directions:

1. In a bowl, mix the flour with the cocoa, the egg, and the other ingredients and whisk really well.

9

2. Preheat the waffle iron to medium-high, pour the chaffle mixture inside, close the waffle iron, cook for 5 minutes, transfer to a plate and serve.

Nutrition: **Calories**: 251; **Fat**: 22.1g; **Fiber**: 1.2g; **Carbs**: 4g; **Protein**: 12g

2. CREAMY CHAFFLE

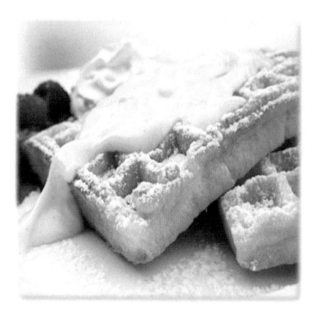

Servings: 2

Preparation Time: 5 Minutes

Cooking Time: 5 Minutes

Ingredients:

- ✓ 1 egg, whisked
- ✓ 2 tablespoons stevia
- ✓ 1 tablespoon heavy cream
- ✓ ½ teaspoon almond extract
- ✓ 1 teaspoon almond flour
- ✓ ½ teaspoon baking soda

Directions:

1. In a bowl, mix the egg with the cream, Stevia, and the other ingredients and whisk well.

2. Preheat the waffle iron at medium-high, pour half of the batter, close the iron, cook the chaffle for 4 minutes and transfer to a plate.

3. Repeat with the rest of the batter and serve warm.

Nutrition: **Calories**: 66; **Fat**: 4.5 g; **Fiber**: 1g; **Carbs**: 2 g; **Protein**: 7.4 g

3. BERRY CHAFFLE

💗 **Servings:** 2

🍪 **Preparation Time:** 5 Minutes

⏰ **Cooking Time:** 5 Minutes

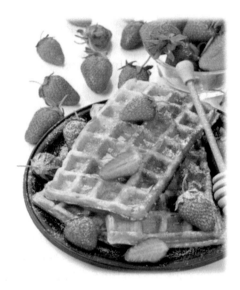

Ingredients:

- ✓ 1 egg, whisked
- ✓ 2 tablespoons stevia
- ✓ 1 teaspoon coconut flour
- ✓ 4 Strawberries, chopped
- ✓ ½ teaspoon baking powder
- ✓ 1 teaspoon cream cheese, soft

Directions:

1. In a bowl, mix the berries with the egg, Stevia, and the other ingredients and whisk well.

2. Heat up the waffle iron over medium-high heat, pour half of the batter, close the waffle maker, cook for 5 minutes and transfer to a plate.

3. Repeat with the other half of the batter and serve the chaffles warm.

Nutrition: **Calories:** 58; **Fat:** 5 g; **Fiber:** 1.2 g; **Carbs:** 2 g; **Protein:** 3.2 g

4. PUMPKIN CHAFFLE

💗 **Servings:** 2

🍪 **Preparation Time:** 5 Minutes

⏰ **Cooking Time:** 5 Minutes

Ingredients:

- ✓ ½ cup mozzarella cheese, shredded
- ✓ 1 tablespoon coconut flour
- ✓ 1 egg, whisked
- ✓ 1 tablespoon stevia
- ✓ 2 tablespoons pumpkin puree
- ✓ 2 tablespoons cream cheese
- ✓ ½ teaspoon almond extract

Directions:

1. In a bowl, mix the mozzarella with the flour, egg, and the other ingredients and whisk well.

2. Heat up the waffle iron over high heat, pour half of the batter, close the waffle maker, cook for 5 minutes and transfer to a plate.

3. Repeat with the other part of the batter and serve the chaffles warm.

Nutrition: Calories: 200; **Fat:** 15g; **Fiber:** 1.2g; **Carbs:** 3.4g; **Protein:** 12.05g

5. CINNAMON CHAFFLE

❤ **Servings:** 1

 Preparation Time: 5 Minutes

⏱ **Cooking Time**: 5 Minutes

Ingredients:

- ✓ Cooking spray
- ✓ 2 ounces cream cheese, soft
- ✓ 1 egg, whisked
- ✓ 2 teaspoons monk fruit sweetener
- ✓ 1 teaspoon coconut flour
- ✓ 2 teaspoons cinnamon powder
- ✓ ½ teaspoon baking soda

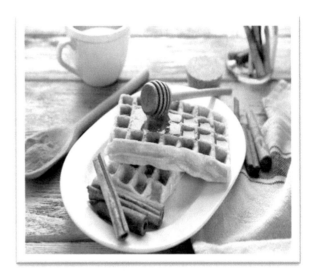

Directions:

1. In a bowl, mix the cream cheese with the egg and the other ingredients except for the cooking spray and whisk well.

2. Grease the waffle iron with the cooking spray, pour the batter, spread, close the waffle maker, cook for 5 minutes, transfer to a plate and serve.

Nutrition: Calories: 121; **Fat:** 8.4g; **Fiber:** 2.3g; **Carbs:** 4g; **Protein:** 2.3g

6. SIMPLE PIZZA CHAFFLE

♥ **Servings:** 2

Preparation Time: 10 Minutes

⏱ **Cooking Time:** 5 Minutes

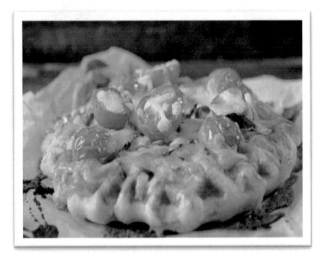

Ingredients:

- ✓ 1 egg, whisked
- ✓ ½ teaspoon Italian seasoning
- ✓ ½ cup mozzarella cheese, shredded
- ✓ 1 tablespoon tomato paste

Directions:

1. In a bowl, mix the egg with half of the cheese and Italian seasoning and stir well.

2. Preheat the waffle iron over medium-high heat, add half of the chaffle mix, spread, close the waffle maker, and cook for 5 minutes.

3. Repeat with the remaining batter, spread the tomato passata over each chaffle, and serve.

> **Nutrition:** **Calories**: 254; **Fat:** 12.3g; **Fiber:** 3.4g; **Carbs:** 4g; **Protein:** 11g

7. HERBED PIZZA CHAFFLE

♥ **Servings:** 2

Preparation Time: 5 Minutes

⏱ **Cooking Time:** 8 Minutes

Ingredients:

- ✓ 1 egg, whisked
- ✓ ½ teaspoon oregano, dried
- ✓ ½ teaspoon basil, dried
- ✓ ½ teaspoon parsley flakes
- ✓ ½ teaspoon garlic powder
- ✓ 2 tablespoons tomato passata
- ✓ 1 cup mozzarella shredded, shredded

Directions:

1. In a bowl, mix the egg with the herbs and half of the mozzarella and stir well.

2. Preheat the waffle iron over medium-high heat, pour half of the chaffle mix, cook for 4 minutes and transfer to a plate.

3. Repeat with the rest of the batter, spread the tomato passata and the rest of the cheese over the chaffles, and serve.

Nutrition: **Calories**: 252; **Fat**: 11g; **Fiber**: 3.2g; **Carbs**: 5g; **Protein**: 11.2g

8. SPINACH PIZZA CHAFFLE

💕 **Servings**: 2

🍰 **Preparation Time**: 5 Minutes

⏰ **Cooking Time**: 6 Minutes

Ingredients:

- ✓ 1 egg, whisked
- ✓ ½ cup mozzarella, shredded
- ✓ 1 tablespoon cheddar, shredded
- ✓ 2 tablespoons cream cheese, soft
- ✓ 1 teaspoon onion powder
- ✓ ¼ cup spinach, torn
- ✓ ½ teaspoon garlic powder
- ✓ 2 tablespoons tomato passata

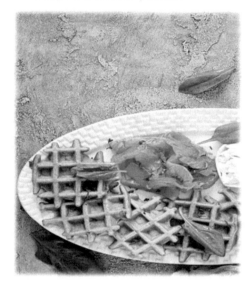

Directions:

1. In a bowl, mix the eggs with the mozzarella and the other ingredients except for the cheddar, spinach, and passata, then stir.

2. Preheat the waffle iron over medium-high heat, pour half of the chaffle mix, cook for 6 minutes and transfer to a plate.

3. Repeat with the rest of the batter spread the remaining ingredients over the chaffles, and serve.

Nutrition: **Calories**: 252; **Fat**: 8.3g; **Fiber**: 4.2g; **Carbs**: 5g; **Protein**: 11.2g

9. ROASTED PEPPERS PIZZA CHAFFLE

💗 **Servings**: 2

🧇 **Preparation Time**: 5 Minutes

⏱ **Cooking Time**: 5 Minutes

Ingredients:

- ✓ 1 egg, whisked
- ✓ ½ cup cheddar cheese, shredded
- ✓ ¼ cup roasted peppers, chopped
- ✓ ½ teaspoon oregano, dried
- ✓ ½ teaspoon garlic powder
- ✓ 2 tablespoons tomato passata

Directions:

1. In a bowl, mix the egg with the cheese and the ingredients except for the peppers and passata and stir.

2. Preheat the waffle iron over high heat, pour half of the chaffle mix, cook for 5 minutes and transfer to a plate.

3. Repeat with the rest of the batter; spread the remaining ingredients over the chaffles, and serve.

Nutrition: Calories: 202g; **Fat**: 12.3g; **Fiber**: 4.2g; **Carbs**: 5g; **Protein**: 11.2g

10. MUSHROOM CHAFFLE

💗 **Servings**: 2

🧇 **Preparation Time**: 5 Minutes

⏱ **Cooking Time**: 6 Minutes

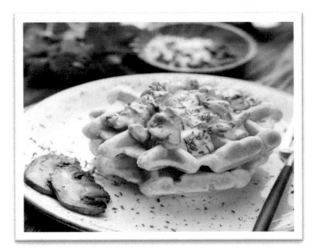

Ingredients:

- ✓ 2 eggs, whisked
- ✓ ½ cup mozzarella, shredded
- ✓ ½ cup mushrooms, sliced
- ✓ 1 teaspoon coriander, ground
- ✓ ½ teaspoon rosemary, dried
- ✓ ½ teaspoon cayenne pepper
- ✓ 2 tablespoons tomato passata

Directions:

1. In a bowl, mix the eggs with mozzarella, coriander, rosemary, and cayenne and stir well.

2. Preheat the waffle iron over medium-

high heat, pour half of the chaffle mix, cook for 6 minutes and transfer to a plate.

3. Repeat with the rest of the batter, spread the passata and the mushrooms over the chaffles, and serve.

Directions:

1. In a bowl, mix the eggs with the milk, oil, and the other ingredients and whisk well.

2. Preheat the waffle iron, pour 1/6 of the batter, cook for 8 minutes and transfer to a plate.

3. Repeat with the rest of the batter and serve.

11. JALAPENO CHAFFLE

💜 Servings: 2

⬛ Preparation Time: 5 Minutes

⏰ Cooking Time: 10 Minutes

Ingredients:

- ✓ 2 eggs, whisked
- ✓ 2 cups almond milk
- ✓ 2 tablespoons avocado oil
- ✓ ½ cup cheddar, shredded
- ✓ 1 cup almond flour
- ✓ 1 tablespoon baking powder
- ✓ A pinch of salt and black pepper
- ✓ ½ teaspoon garlic powder
- ✓ 2 Jalapenos, minced

12. GREEN CHILI CHAFFLE

💜 Servings: 2

⬛ Preparation Time: 10 Minutes

⏰ Cooking Time: 10 Minutes

Ingredients:

- ✓ 2 eggs, whisked
- ✓ 1 and ½ cup almond flour
- ✓ ½ cup cream cheese, soft
- ✓ ½ cup almond milk
- ✓ 1 teaspoon baking soda
- ✓ A pinch of salt and black k pepper
- ✓ ½ cup green chilies, minced

✓ 1 tablespoon chives, chopped

Directions:

1. In a bowl, mix the eggs with the flour, cream cheese, and the other ingredients and whisk.

2. Preheat the waffle iron, pour 1/6 of the batter, close the waffle maker, cook for 8 minutes and transfer to a plate.

3. Repeat with the rest of the batter and serve.

Nutrition: **Calories**: 265; **Fat**: 7; **Fiber**: 3

Carbs: 5.4; **Protein**: 6

13. HOT PORK CHAFFLES

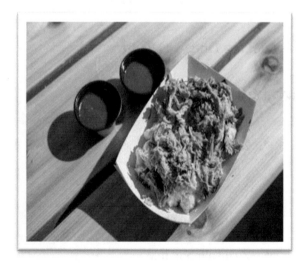

♥ **Servings:** 2

Preparation Time: 10 Minutes

⏰ **Cooking Time**: 10 Minutes

Ingredients:

✓ 1 cup pulled pork, cooked

✓ 2 tablespoons parmesan, grated

✓ 2 eggs, whisked

✓ 2 red chilies, minced

✓ 1 cup almond milk

✓ 1 cup almond flour

✓ 2 tablespoons coconut oil, melted

✓ 1 teaspoon baking powder

Directions:

1. In a bowl, mix the pulled pork with the eggs, parmesan, and the other ingredients and whisk well.

2. Heat up the waffle maker, pour ¼ of the chaffle mix, cook for 8 minutes and transfer to a plate.

3. Repeat with the rest of the mix and serve.

Nutrition: **Calories**: 300; **Fat**: 13g; **Fiber**: 4g

Carbs: 7.2g; **Protein**: 15g

14. SPICY CHICKEN CHAFFLES

💜 **Servings**: 2

🍫 **Preparation Time**: 10 Minutes

⏰ **Cooking Time**: 10 Minutes

Ingredients:

- ✓ 2 eggs, whisked
- ✓ 1 cup rotisserie chicken, skinless, boneless, and shredded
- ✓ 1 cup mozzarella, shredded
- ✓ ½ cup milk
- ✓ 2 teaspoons chili powder
- ✓ 1 teaspoon sriracha sauce
- ✓ 1 tablespoon chives, chopped
- ✓ ½ teaspoon baking powder

Directions:

1. In a bowl, mix the eggs with the chicken, mozzarella, and the other ingredients and whisk.

2. Preheat the waffle maker, pour ¼ of the batter, cook for 10 minutes, and transfer to a plate.

3. Repeat with the rest of the batter and serve.

Nutrition: **Calories**: 320; **Fat**: 8g; **Fiber**: 2g

Carbs: 5.3g; **Protein**: 12g

15. SPICY RICOTTA CHAFFLES

💜 **Servings**: 2

🍫 **Preparation Time**: 10 Minutes

⏰ **Cooking Time**: 10 Minutes

Ingredients:

- ✓ 2 cups coconut flour
- ✓ 1 and ½ cups coconut milk
- ✓ 2 tablespoons olive oil
- ✓ A pinch of salt and black pepper
- ✓ ½ cup ricotta cheese
- ✓ 1 teaspoon baking powder
- ✓ 2 eggs, whisked
- ✓ ½ cup chives, chopped
- ✓ 1 Red chili pepper, minced
- ✓ 1 Jalapeno, chopped

Directions:

1. In a bowl, mix the flour with the milk, oil, and the other ingredients and whisk well.

2. Heat up the waffle iron, pour ¼ of the batter, cook for 10 minutes and transfer to a plate.

3. Repeat with the rest of the chaffle mix and serve.

Nutrition: **Calories**: 262; **Fat**: 8g; **Fiber**: 2.4g; **Carbs**: 3.2g; **Protein**: 8g

16. KETO CHOCOLATE TWINKIE COPYCAT CHAFFLE

❤ **Servings:** 2

🧇 **Preparation Time:** 5 Minutes

⏰ **Cooking Time:** 12 Minutes

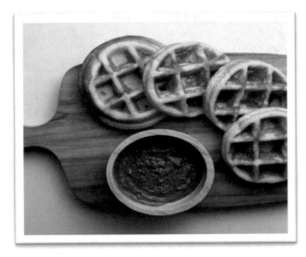

Ingredients:

- ✓ 2 tablespoons of butter (cooled)
- ✓ 2 oz. Cream cheese softened
- ✓ Two large egg room temperature
- ✓ 1 teaspoon of vanilla essence
- ✓ 1/4 cup Lakanto confectionery
- ✓ A pinch of pink salt
- ✓ 1/4 cup almond flour
- ✓ 2 tablespoons coconut powder
- ✓ 2 tablespoons cocoa powder
- ✓ 1 teaspoon baking powder

Directions:

1. Preheat the Maker of Corndog.

2. Melt the butter for a minute and let it cool.

3. In the butter, whisk the eggs until smooth.

4. Remove sugar, cinnamon, sweetener and blend well.

5. Add almond flour, coconut flour, cacao powder, and baking powder.

6. Blend until well embedded.

7. Fill each well with two tablespoons of batter and spread evenly.

8. Close the lid and let it cook for 4 minutes.

9. Lift from the rack and cool it down.

Nutrition: **Calories:** 104; **Total Fat:** 6.2g

Cholesterol: 67.1mg; **Sodium:** 485.5mg;

Total Carbohydrates: 5.3g; **Dietary Fiber:** 1.7g;

Sugars: 1.6g; **Protein:** 4.4g; **Vitamin A:** 80.1μg;

Vitamin C: 0mg

17. KETO CHAFFLE STUFFING

♥ **Servings:** 2

Preparation Time: 20 Minutes

⏱ **Cooking Time**: 40 Minutes

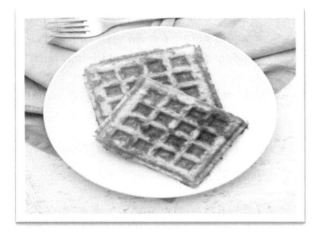

Ingredients: -Basic   chaffle
ingredients:

- ✓ 1/2 cup cheese mozzarella, cheddar cheese, or a combination of both
- ✓ 2 eggs
- ✓ 1/4 teaspoon of garlic powder
- ✓ 1/2 teaspoon onion powder
- ✓ 1/2 teaspoon dried chicken seasoning
- ✓ 1/4 teaspoon salt
- ✓ 1/4 teaspoon pepper

Ingredients: -for filling:

- ✓ 1 Diced onion
- ✓ 2 Celery stems
- ✓ 4 oz. Mushrooms diced
- ✓ 4 cups of butter for sautéing
- ✓ 3 eggs

Directions:

1. First, make a chaffle. This recipe makes four mini-chaffles.

2. Preheat the mini waffle iron.

3. Preheat oven to 350°F

4. In a medium bowl, mix the chaffle ingredients.

5. Pour 1/4 of the mixture into a mini waffle maker and cook each chaffle for about four minutes.

6. Once cooked, set them aside.

7. In a small skillet, fry the onions, celery, and mushrooms until soft.

8. In a separate bowl, split the chaffle into small pieces and add sautéed vegetables and three eggs. Mix until the ingredients are completely bonded.

9. Add the mixture of fillings to a small casserole dish (about 4x4) and bake at 350 degrees for about 30-40 minutes.

Note: Make four chaffles.

Nutrition: **Calories**: 229; **Total Fat**: 17.6g

Cholesterol: 265.6mg; **Sodium**: 350mg

Total Carbohydrates: 4.6g; **Dietary Fiber**: 1.1g

Sugars: 2g; **Protein**: 13.7g; **Vitamin A**: 217.2µg

Vitamin C: 2.4mg

18. KETO CORNBREAD CHAFFLE

Servings: 2

Preparation Time: 5 Minutes

Cooking Time: 5 Minutes

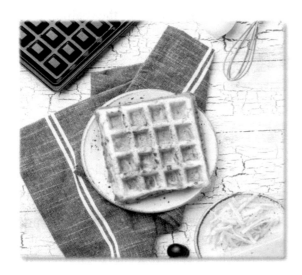

Ingredients:

- ✓ 1 egg

- ✓ 1/2 cup shredded cheddar cheese (or mozzarella cheese)

- ✓ 5 Slices Jalapeno (optional) freshly picked or fresh

- ✓ 1 teaspoon of Frank's Red-Hot Sauce

- ✓ 1/4 teaspoon corn extract as an essential secret ingredient!

- ✓ A pinch of salt

Directions:

1. Preheat the Mini waffle maker, place the eggs in a small bowl.

2. Add the remaining ingredients and combine until well absorbed.

3. Apply one tablespoon of shredded cheese to the waffle maker for 30 seconds before removing the mixture. It produces a very clean and friendly crust!

4. Add half of the mixture to the preheated waffle maker.

5. Cook for a total of 3-4 minutes. The more they remain, the crunchier.

6. Enjoy it served warm!

Nutrition: **Calories:** 150; **Total Fat:** 11.8g

Cholesterol: 121mg; **Sodium:** 1399.4mg

Total Carbohydrates: 1.1g; **Dietary Fiber:** 0g

Sugars: 0.2g; **Protein:** 9.6g; **Vitamin A:** 134.1µg

Vitamin C: 0.1mg

19. MAPLE PUMPKIN KETO CHAFFLE

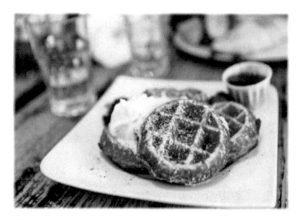

❤️ **Servings:** 2

🧇 **Preparation Time**: 5 Minutes

⏰ **Cooking Time**: 4 Minutes

Ingredients:

- ✓ 3/4 teaspoon baking powder
- ✓ 2 eggs
- ✓ 4 teaspoons heavy whipping cream
- ✓ 1/2 cup mozzarella cheese, shredded
- ✓ 2 teaspoons Liquid Stevia
- ✓ A pinch of salt
- ✓ 3/4 teaspoons pumpkin pie spice
- ✓ 1 teaspoon coconut flour
- ✓ 2 teaspoons pumpkin puree (100% pumpkin)
- ✓ 1/2 teaspoons vanilla

Directions:

1. Preheat the mini waffle maker until hot

2. Whisk the egg in a bowl, add cheese, and then mix well

3. Stir in the remaining ingredients (except toppings, if any).

4. Scoop 1/2 of the batter onto the waffle maker, spread across evenly

5. Cook 3-4 minutes, until done as desired (or crispy).

6. Gently remove from the waffle maker and let it cool

7. Repeat with the remaining batter.

8. Top with sugar-free maple syrup or keto ice cream.

9. Serve and Enjoy!

Nutrition: **Calories:** 201; **Net carbs:** 2g

Fat: 15g; **Protein**: 12g

20. KETO ALMOND BLUEBERRY CHAFFLE

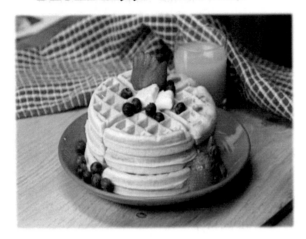

♥ **Servings:** 2 Chaffles

Preparation Time: 5 Minutes

⏰ **Cooking Time**: 5 Minutes

Ingredients:

- ✓ 1 teaspoon baking powder
- ✓ 2 eggs
- ✓ 1 cup of mozzarella cheese
- ✓ 2 tablespoons almond flour
- ✓ 3 tablespoons blueberries
- ✓ 1 teaspoon cinnamon
- ✓ 2 teaspoons of Swerve

Directions:

1. Preheat the mini waffle maker until hot
2. Whisk egg in a bowl, add cheese, and then mix well
3. Stir in the remaining ingredients (except toppings, if any).
4. Grease the preheated waffle maker with non-stick cooking spray.
5. Scoop 1/2 of the batter onto the waffle maker, spread across evenly
6. Cook until a bit browned and crispy, about 4 minutes.
7. Cook 3-4 minutes, until done as desired (or crispy).
8. Gently remove from the waffle maker and let it cool
9. Repeat with the remaining batter.
10. Top with keto syrup
11. Serve and Enjoy!

Nutrition: **Calories**: 116; **Net carbs**: 1g **Fat**: 8g; **Protein**: 8g

21. KETO BREAKFAST CHAFFLE

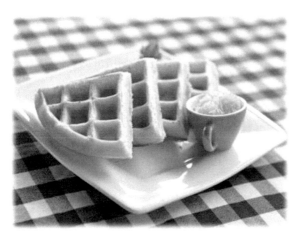

🖤 **Servings**: 1

🧇 **Preparation Time**: 3 Minutes

⏰ **Cooking Time**: 6 Minutes

Ingredients:

- ✓ 2 tablespoons butter
- ✓ 1 egg
- ✓ 1/2 cup Monterey Jack Cheese
- ✓ 1 tablespoon almond flour

Directions:

1. Preheat the mini waffle maker until hot
2. Whisk the egg in a bowl, add cheese, and then mix well
3. Stir in the remaining ingredients (except toppings, if any).
4. Grease the waffle maker and Scoop 1/2 of the batter onto the waffle maker, spread across evenly
5. Cook until a bit browned and crispy, about 4 minutes.
6. Gently remove from the waffle maker and let it cool
7. Repeat with the remaining batter.
8. Melt butter in a pan. Add chaffles to the pan and cook for 2 minutes on each side
9. Remove from the pan and let it cool.
10. Serve and Enjoy!

Nutrition: **Calories**: 257; **Net carbs**: 1g; **Fat**: 24g; **Protein**: 11g

22. SWEET CINNAMON "SUGAR" CHAFFLE

🖤 **Servings**: 1

🧇 **Preparation Time**: 5 Minutes

⏰ **Cooking Time**: 4 Minutes

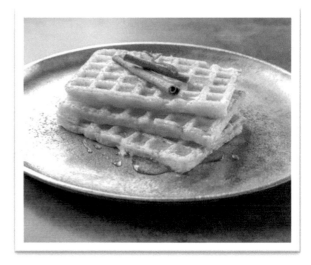

24

Ingredients:

- ✓ 1/2 teaspoon cinnamon (topping)
- ✓ 10 Drops of liquid Stevia
- ✓ 1 tablespoon almond flour
- ✓ Two large eggs
- ✓ A splash of vanilla
- ✓ 1/2 cup mozzarella cheese

Directions:

1. Preheat the waffle maker until hot
2. Whisk egg in a bowl, add cheese, and then mix well
3. Stir in the remaining ingredients (except toppings, if any).
4. Scoop 1/2 of the batter onto the waffle maker, spread across evenly
5. Cook 3-4 minutes, until done as desired (or crispy).
6. Gently remove from the waffle maker and let it cool
7. Repeat with the remaining batter.
8. Top with melted butter and a sprinkle of cinnamon.
9. Serve and Enjoy!

Nutrition: Calories: 221; **Net carbs**: 2g; **Fat**: 17g; **Protein**: 12g

23. KETO "CINNAMON ROLL" CHAFFLES

💗 **Servings:** 2

🧇 **Preparation Time**: 5 Minutes

⏰ **Cooking Time**: 10 Minutes

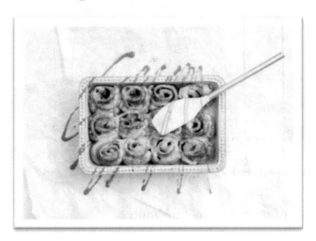

Ingredients: Cinnamon Roll Chaffle:

- ✓ 1/2 cup mozzarella cheese
- ✓ 1/4 teaspoon baking powder
- ✓ 1 teaspoon Granulated Swerve
- ✓ 1 tablespoon almond flour
- ✓ 1 teaspoon cinnamon
- ✓ 1 egg

Cinnamon Roll Swirl:

- ✓ 2 teaspoons confectioners swerve
- ✓ 1 tablespoon butter
- ✓ 1 teaspoon cinnamon

Keto Cinnamon Roll Glaze:

- ✓ 2 teaspoons swerve confectioners
- ✓ 1/4 teaspoons vanilla extract
- ✓ 1 tablespoon cream cheese
- ✓ 1 tablespoon butter

Directions:

1. Preheat the waffle maker until hot

2. Add Cinnamon roll chaffle ingredients in a bowl and combine well

3. In another small bowl, add the cinnamon Roll Swirl ingredients, and stir well.

4. Microwave for 15 seconds and mix well.

5. Spray the waffle maker with non-stick spray and add 1/3 of the batter to your waffle maker.

6. Swirl in 1/3 of the "cinnamon roll swirl ingredients" mixture on top of it.

7. Cook for 3-4 minutes. Repeat for the remaining batter.

8. In a small bowl, add "Keto cinnamon roll glaze ingredients," combine and microwave for 20 seconds.

9. Drizzle on top of the chaffles

Nutrition: **Calories:** 180; **Net carbs**: 1g; **Fat**: 16g; **Protein**: 7g

24. SWEET & SAVORY MILKY CHAFFLE

💙 **Servings:** 2

🍳 **Preparation Time**: 5 Minutes

⏰ **Cooking Time:** 4 Minutes

Ingredients:

- ✓ 3/4 teaspoon baking powder
- ✓ 2 eggs
- ✓ 4 teaspoon heavy whipping cream
- ✓ 1/2 cup coconut milk
- ✓ 1/2 cup mozzarella cheese, shredded
- ✓ 10 Drops Liquid Stevia
- ✓ 1 teaspoon coconut or almond flour
- ✓ 1/2 teaspoon vanilla

Directions:

1. Preheat the mini waffle maker until hot

2. Whisk the eggs in a bowl, add cheese, and then mix well

3. Stir in the remaining ingredients (except toppings, if any).

4. Scoop 1/2 of the batter onto the waffle maker, spread across evenly.

5. Cook 3-4 minutes, until done as desired

(or crispy).

6. Gently remove from the waffle maker and let it cool

7. Repeat with the remaining batter.

8. Top with coconut milk and whipping cream.

9. Serve and Enjoy!

Nutrition: Calories: 231; **Net carbs:** 2g; **Fat:** 21g; **Protein:** 12g

25. SWEET RASPBERRY CHAFFLE

💗 **Servings:** 2

🧇 **Preparation Time:** 5 Minutes

⏰ **Cooking Time:** 5 Minutes

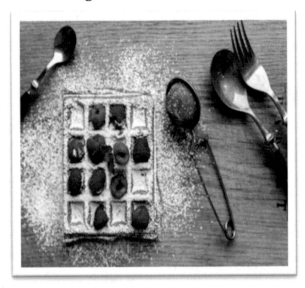

Ingredients:

- ✓ 1 teaspoon baking powder
- ✓ 2 eggs
- ✓ 1 cup of mozzarella cheese
- ✓ 2 tablespoons almond flour
- ✓ 4 Raspberries, chopped
- ✓ 1 teaspoon cinnamon
- ✓ 10 Drops Stevia, liquid

Directions:

1. Preheat the mini waffle maker until hot

2. Whisk egg in a bowl, add cheese, and then mix well

3. Stir in the remaining ingredients (except toppings, if any).

4. Grease the preheated waffle maker with non-stick cooking spray.

5. Scoop 1/2 of the batter onto the waffle maker, spread across evenly

6. Cook until a bit browned and crispy, about 4 minutes.

7. Cook 3-4 minutes, until done as desired (or crispy).

8. Gently remove from the waffle maker and let it cool

9. Repeat with the remaining batter.

10. Top with keto syrup

11. Serve and Enjoy!

Nutrition: Calories: 116; **Net carbs:** 1g; **Fat:** 8g; **Protein:** 8g

26. SAVORY & CRISPY BREAKFAST CHAFFLE

💟 **Servings:** 1

🍫 **Preparation Time**: 3 Minutes

⏰ **Cooking Time:** 6 Minutes

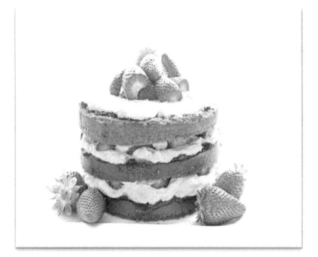

Ingredients:

- ✓ 2 tablespoons butter
- ✓ 1 egg
- ✓ 1/2 cup Monterey Jack Cheese
- ✓ 1 tablespoon almond flour

Directions:

1. Preheat the mini waffle maker until hot
2. Whisk the egg in a bowl, add cheese, and then mix well
3. Stir in the remaining ingredients (except toppings, if any).
4. Grease waffle maker and Scoop 1/2 of the batter onto the waffle maker, spread across evenly
5. Cook until a bit browned and crispy, about 4 minutes.
6. Gently remove from the waffle maker and let it cool
7. Repeat with the remaining batter.
8. Melt butter in a pan. Add chaffles to the pan and cook for 2 minutes on each side
9. Remove from the pan and let it cool.
10. Serve and Enjoy!

Nutrition: **Calories**: 257; **Net carbs**: 1g; **Fat**: 24g; **Protein**: 11g

---

27. STRAWBERRY SHORTCAKE CHAFFLE

💟 **Servings:** 2 Chaffles

🍫 **Preparation Time**: 4 Minutes

⏰ **Cooking Time**: 12 Minutes

Ingredients:

Strawberry topping:

- ✓ 3 Fresh strawberries
- ✓ 1/2 tablespoons granulated swerve

Sweet Chaffle Ingredients:

- ✓ 1 tablespoon granulated swerve
- ✓ Keto Whipped Cream
- ✓ 1 tablespoon almond flour
- ✓ 1/2 cup mozzarella cheese
- ✓ 1/4 teaspoon vanilla extract
- ✓ 1 egg

Directions:

1. Preheat the waffle maker until hot
2. Whisk the egg in a bowl, add cheese and then mix well
3. In a small bowl, add the strawberries and swerve, mix until well-combined. Set aside.
4. In another bowl, add the "sweet chaffle ingredients" and mix thoroughly.
5. Pour 1/3 of the batter into your mini waffle maker and cook for 3-4 minutes.
6. Rove gently and set aside to cool
7. Repeat for the remaining batter, make three chaffle cakes in total.
8. Assemble the Chaffle by topping with strawberries and whipped cream.
9. Serve and Enjoy!

Nutrition: **Calories**: 112; **Net carbs**: 1g; **Fat**: 8g; **Protein**: 7g

28. KETO CHAFFLE TACO SHELLS

Servings: 2

Preparation Time: 5 Minutes

Cooking Time: 20 Minutes

Ingredients:

- ✓ 1 tablespoon almond flour
- ✓ 2 eggs
- ✓ 1/4 teaspoon taco seasoning
- ✓ 1 cup taco blend cheese

Directions:

1. Preheat the mini waffle maker until hot
2. Add ingredients to a bowl and mix well
3. Grease waffle maker with cooking spray
4. Add 1-2 tablespoons of batter at a time to the waffle maker.
5. Cook for about 4 minutes.

6. Gently remove from the waffle maker and drape over the side of a bowl or pie pan. Repeat with the remaining batter.

7. Remove from the pan and let it cool.

8. Fill taco shells with favorite toppings

9. Serve and enjoy!

> **Nutrition:** **Calories**: 113; **Net carbs**: 1g; **Fat**: 9g; **Protein:** 8g

29. MINI KETO PIZZA CHAFFLE

❤ **Servings:** 2

▦ **Preparation Time**: 5Minutes

⏰ **Cooking Time**: 10 Minutes

Ingredients:

- ✓ 1/4 teaspoon basil
- ✓ 2 tablespoons mozzarella cheese
- ✓ 2 tablespoons low carb pasta sauce
- ✓ 1 tablespoon almond flour
- ✓ 1/4 teaspoon garlic powder
- ✓ 1 egg
- ✓ 1/2 cup shredded mozzarella cheese
- ✓ 1/2 teaspoon baking powder

Directions:

1. Preheat the mini waffle maker until hot

2. Add all ingredients except the pasta sauce to a bowl and mix well.

3. Grease the waffle maker and put half of the batter spread across evenly.

4. Cook until completely done, about 4 minutes.

5. Gently remove from the waffle maker and let it cool.

6. Repeat with the remaining batter.

7. Once they are cooked, place them on the lined baking sheet in the toaster oven.

8. Top each pizza crust with one tablespoon of pasta sauce each.

9. Sprinkle with one tablespoon each of shredded mozzarella cheese.

10. Bake at 350°F for 5 minutes until the cheese is a little melted.

11. Remove from the oven and let it cool.

12. Serve and Enjoy!

> **Nutrition:** **Calories**: 195; **Net carbs**: 2g; **Fat**: 14g**Protein:** 13g

Chapter 2. Special Chaffle Recipes

30. BREAKFAST FESTIVE CHAFFLE SANDWICH

💗 **Servings:** 2

🧇 **Preparation Time:** 10 Minutes

⏰ **Cooking Time:** 10 Minutes

Ingredients:

- ✓ 2 Basics cooked chaffles
- ✓ Cooking spray
- ✓ 2 slices bacon
- ✓ 1 egg

Directions:

1. Spray your pan with oil.
2. Place it over medium heat.
3. Cook the bacon until golden and crispy.
4. Put the bacon on top of one chaffle.
5. In the same pan, cook the egg without mixing until the yolk is set.
6. Add the egg on top of the bacon.
7. Top with another chaffle.

31. COOKIE DOUGH CHAFFLE

💗 **Servings:** 2

🧇 **Preparation Time:** 5 Minutes

⏰ **Cooking Time:** 7-9 Minutes

Ingredients: For the Batter:

- ✓ 4 eggs
- ✓ ¼ cup heavy cream
- ✓ 1 teaspoon vanilla extract
- ✓ ¼ cup stevia
- ✓ 6 tablespoons coconut flour
- ✓ 1 teaspoon baking powder
- ✓ A pinch of salt
- ✓ ¼ cup unsweetened chocolate chips

Other:

- ✓ 2 tablespoons cooking spray to brush the waffle maker

✓ ¼ cup heavy cream, whipped

Directions:

1. Preheat the waffle maker.

2. Introduce the eggs and heavy cream to a bowl and stir in the vanilla extract, Stevia, coconut flour, baking powder, and salt. Mix until just combined.

3. Stir in the chocolate chips and combine.

4. Brush the heated waffle maker with cooking spray and add a few tablespoons of the batter.

5. Cover and cook for about 7–8 minutes, depending on your waffle maker.

6. Serve with whipped cream on top.

Nutrition: **Calories**: 3; **Fat**: 32.3g; **Carbs**: 12.6g

Sugar: 0.5; **Protein**: 9g; **Sodium**: 117mg

32. THANKSGIVING PUMPKIN SPICE CHAFFLE

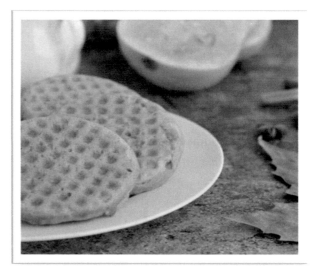

💜 **Servings**: 2

🧇 **Preparation Time**: 5 Minutes

⏰ **Cooking Time**: 5 Minutes

Ingredients:

✓ 1 cup egg whites

✓ ¼ cup pumpkin puree

✓ 2 teaspoons. Pumpkin pie spice

✓ 2 teaspoons. Coconut flour

✓ ½ teaspoon vanilla

✓ 1 teaspoon baking powder

✓ 1 teaspoon baking soda

✓ 1/8 teaspoon cinnamon powder

✓ 1 cup mozzarella cheese, grated

✓ 1/2 teaspoon garlic powder

Directions:

1. Switch on your square waffle maker. Spray with non-stick spray.

2. Beat egg whites until fluffy and white.

3. Add pumpkin puree, pumpkin pie spice, and coconut flour to the egg whites and beat again.

4. Stir in the cheese, cinnamon powder, garlic powder, baking soda, and powder.

5. Pour half of the batter into the waffle maker.

6. Close the maker and cook for about three minutes.

7. Repeat with the remaining batter.

8. Remove chaffles from the maker.

9. Serve hot and enjoy!

Nutrition: **Protein**: 51%; **Fat**: 41%;

Carbohydrates: 8%

33. PUMPKIN SPICE CHAFFLES

♥ **Servings**: 2

Preparation Time: 10 Minutes

Cooking Time: 14 Minutes

Ingredients:

✓ 1 egg, beaten

✓ ½ teaspoon pumpkin pie spice

✓ ½ cup finely grated mozzarella cheese

✓ 1 tablespoon sugar-free pumpkin puree

Directions:

1. Preheat the waffle iron.

2. In a bowl, add all the ingredients.

3. Open the iron, pour in half of the batter, close, and cook until crispy, 6 to 7 minutes.

4. Remove the chaffle onto a plate and set it aside.

5. Make another chaffle with the remaining batter.

6. Allow cooling and serve afterward.

Nutrition: **Calories**: 90; **Fats**: 6.46g; **Carbs**: 1.98g; **Net Carbs**: 1.58g; **Protein**: 5.94g

34. CHAFFLE FRUIT SNACKS

💟 **Servings:** 2

🧇 **Preparation Time**: 10 Minutes

⏰ **Cooking Time**: 14 Minutes

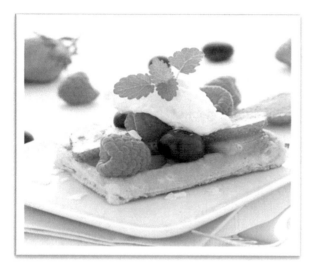

Ingredients:

- ✓ 1 egg, beaten
- ✓ ½ cup finely grated cheddar cheese
- ✓ ½ cup Greek yogurt for topping
- ✓ 8 Raspberries and blackberries for topping

Directions:

1. Preheat the waffle iron.

2. Mix the egg and cheddar cheese in a medium bowl.

3. Open the iron and add half of the mixture. Close and cook until crispy, 7 minutes.

4. Remove the chaffle onto a plate and make another with the remaining mixture.

5. Cut each chaffle into wedges and arrange it on a plate.

6. Top each waffle with a tablespoon of yogurt and then two berries.

7. Serve afterward.

Nutrition: **Calories**: 207; **Fats**: 15.29g; **Carbs**: 4.36g; **Net Carbs**: 3.g; **Protein**: 12.91g

35. OPEN-FACED HAM & GREEN BELL PEPPER CHAFFLE SANDWICH

💟 **Servings:** 2

🧇 **Preparation Time**: 10 Minutes

⏰ **Cooking Time**: 10 Minutes

Ingredients:

- ✓ 2 Slices ham
- ✓ Cooking spray
- ✓ 1 green bell pepper, sliced into strips
- ✓ 2 slices cheese
- ✓ 1 tablespoon black olives, pitted and

sliced

- ✓ 2 basic chaffles

Directions:

1. Cook the ham in a pan coated with oil over medium heat.

2. Next, cook the bell pepper.

3. Assemble the open-faced sandwich by topping each chaffle with ham and cheese, bell pepper, and olives.

4. Toast in the oven until the cheese has melted a little.

Nutrition: **Calories**: 36; **Total Fat**: 24.6g

Saturated Fat: 13.6g; **Cholesterol**: 91mg

Sodium: 1154mg; **Potassium**: 440mg

Total Carbohydrates: 8g; **Dietary Fiber**: 2.6g

Protein: 24.5g; **Total Sugars**: 6.3g

36. TACO CHAFFLE

♥ **Servings**: 2

Preparation Time: 8 Minutes

⏲ **Cooking Time**: 20 Minutes

Ingredients:

- ✓ 1 tablespoon olive oil
- ✓ 1 lb. ground beef
- ✓ 1 teaspoon ground cumin
- ✓ 1 teaspoon chili powder
- ✓ ¼ teaspoon onion powder
- ✓ ½ teaspoon garlic powder
- ✓ Salt to taste
- ✓ 4 Basic chaffles
- ✓ 1 cup cabbage, chopped
- ✓ 4 tablespoons salsa (sugar-free)

Directions:

1. Pour the olive oil into a pan over medium heat.

2. Add the ground beef.

3. Season with salt and spices.

4. Cook until brown and crumbly.

5. Fold the chaffle to create a "taco shell."

6. Stuff each chaffle taco with cabbage.

7. Top with ground beef and salsa.

Nutrition: **Calories**: 255; **Total Fat**: 10.9g;

Saturated Fat: 3.2g; **Cholesterol**: 101mg; **Sodium**: 220mg; **Potassium**: 561mg; **Total Carbohydrates**: 3g; **Dietary Fiber**: 1g; **Protein**: 35.1g; **Total Sugars**: 1.3g

37. CHRISTMAS MORNING CHOCO CHAFFLE CAKE

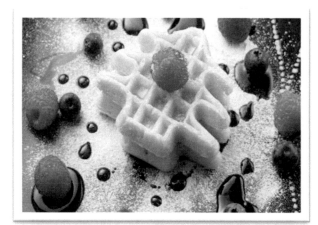

❤️ **Servings:** 2

🧇 **Preparation Time**: 10 Minutes

⏰ **Cooking Time**: 5 Minutes

Ingredients:

- ✓ 8 Keto chocolate square chaffles
- ✓ 2 cups peanut butter
- ✓ 16 oz. Raspberries

Directions:

1. Assemble chaffles in layers.
2. Spread peanut butter in each layer.
3. Top with raspberries.
4. Enjoy cake on Christmas morning with keto coffee!

Nutrition: **Protein**:1; **Fat**:207;

Carbohydrates: 15

38. LT CHAFFLE SANDWICH

❤️ **Servings:** 2

🧇 **Preparation Time**: 10 Minutes

⏰ **Cooking Time**: 15 Minutes

Ingredients:

- ✓ Cooking spray
- ✓ 4 Slices bacon
- ✓ 1 tablespoon mayonnaise
- ✓ 4 Basic chaffles
- ✓ 2 Lettuce leaves
- ✓ 2 Tomato slices

Directions:

1. Coat your pan with foil and place it over medium heat.
2. Cook the bacon until golden and crispy.
3. On top of the chaffle, spread mayo.
4. Top with lettuce, bacon, and tomato.
5. Top with another chaffle.

Nutrition: **Calories**: 238; **Total Fat**: 18.4g

Saturated Fat: 5; **Cholesterol** 44mg; **Sodium:** 931mg; **Potassium**: 258mg; **Total Carbohydrates**: 3g; **Dietary Fiber**: 0.2g; **Protein**: 14.3g; **Total Sugars**: 0.9g

39. MOZZARELLA PEANUT BUTTER CHAFFLE

💔 **Servings:** 2

🧇 **Preparation Time:** 10 Minutes

⏰ **Cooking Time:** 15 Minutes

Ingredients:

- ✓ 1 egg, lightly beaten
- ✓ 2 tablespoons peanut butter
- ✓ 2 tablespoons Swerve
- ✓ 1/2 cup mozzarella cheese, shredded

Directions:

1. Preheat your waffle maker.
2. In a bowl, mix egg, cheese, Swerve, and peanut butter until well combined.
3. Spray waffle maker with cooking spray.
4. Introduce half batter in the hot waffle maker and cook for some minutes or until golden brown. Repeat with the remaining batter.
5. Serve and enjoy.

Nutrition: **Calories:** 150; **Fat:** 11.5; **Carbohydrates:** 5.g; **Sugar:** 1.7; **Protein:** 8.8 **Cholesterol:** 86mg

40. DOUBLE DECKER CHAFFLE

💔 **Servings:** 2

🧇 **Preparation Time:** 7 Minutes

⏰ **Cooking Time:** 10 Minutes

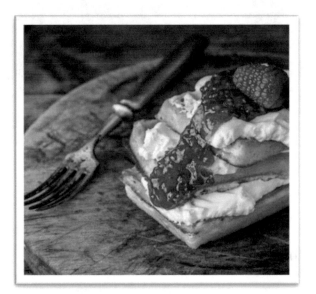

Ingredients:

- ✓ 1 Large egg
- ✓ 1 cup shredded cheese

Topping:

- ✓ 1 Keto chocolate ball
- ✓ 2 oz. Cranberries
- ✓ 2 oz. Blueberries
- ✓ 4 oz. Cranberries puree

Directions:

1. Make 2 minutes dash waffles.

2. Put cranberries and blueberries in the freezer for about hours.

3. For serving, arrange keto chocolate balls between the chaffles.

4. Top with frozen berries,

5. Serve and enjoy!

Nutrition: **Protein:** 78; **Fat:** 223; **Carbohydrates**: 31

41. CINNAMON AND VANILLA CHAFFLE

🐏 **Servings:** 2

🧇 **Preparation Time:** 5 Minutes

⏱ **Cooking Time:** 7-9 Minutes

Ingredients: Batter:

- ✓ 4 eggs
- ✓ 4 Ounces sour cream
- ✓ 1 teaspoon vanilla extract
- ✓ 1 teaspoon cinnamon
- ✓ ¼ cup stevia

- ✓ 5 tablespoons coconut flour

Other:

- ✓ 2 tablespoons coconut oil to brush the waffle maker
- ✓ ½ teaspoon cinnamon for garnishing the chaffles

Directions:

1. Preheat the waffle maker.

2. Add the eggs and sour cream to a bowl and stir with a wire whisk until just combined.

3. Add the vanilla extract, cinnamon, and Stevia and mix until combined.

4. Stir in the coconut flour and stir until combined.

5. Brush the heated waffle maker with coconut oil and add a few tablespoons of the batter.

6. Cover and cook for about 7–8 minutes, depending on your waffle maker.

7. Serve and enjoy.

Nutrition: **Calories:** 224; **Fat:** 11g; **Carbs:** 8.4g; **Sugar:** 0.5; **Protein:** 7.7g; **Sodium:** 77mg

42. CHAFFLES AND ICE-CREAM PLATTER

💟 **Servings:** 2

▨ **Preparation Time**: 10 Minutes

⏲ **Cooking Time**: 5 Minutes

Ingredients:

- ✓ 2 Keto brownie chaffles
- ✓ 2 Scoops vanilla keto ice cream
- ✓ 8 oz. Strawberries, sliced
- ✓ Keto chocolate sauce

Directions:

1. Arrange chaffles, ice cream, strawberries slice in serving plate.
2. Drizzle chocolate sauce on top.
3. Serve and enjoy!

Nutrition: Protein: 26%; **Fat**: 68%; **Carbohydrates**: 6%

43. CHOCO CHIP PUMPKIN CHAFFLE

💟 **Servings:** 2

▨ **Preparation Time**: 10 Minutes

⏲ **Cooking Time**: 15 Minutes

Ingredients:

- ✓ 1 egg, lightly beaten
- ✓ 1 tablespoon almond flour
- ✓ 1 tablespoon unsweetened chocolate chips
- ✓ 1/4 teaspoon pumpkin pie spice
- ✓ 2 tablespoons Swerve
- ✓ 1 tablespoon pumpkin puree
- ✓ 1/2 cup mozzarella cheese, shredded

Directions:

1. Preheat your waffle maker.
2. In a small bowl, mix egg and pumpkin puree.
3. Add pumpkin pie spice, Swerve, almond flour, and cheese and mix well.
4. Stir in chocolate chips.
5. Spray waffle maker with cooking spray.
6. Introduce half batter in the hot waffle maker and cook for 4 minutes. Repeat with the remaining batter.
7. Serve and enjoy.

✓ 6 mushroom slices

✓ 4 teaspoons mayonnaise

✓ 4 large white onion rings

✓ 4 basic chaffles

Directions:

1. Spray your skillet with oil.

2. Place over medium heat.

3. Cook sausage until both sides turn brown

4. Transfer on a plate.

5. Cook the pepperoni and mushrooms for 2 minutes.

6. Spread mayo on the top of the chaffle.

7. Top with the sausage, pepperoni, mushrooms, and onion rings.

8. Top with another chaffle.

44. SAUSAGE & PEPPERONI CHAFFLE SANDWICH

❤️ **Servings:** 2

🧱 **Preparation Time**: 8 Minutes

⏰ **Cooking Time**: 10 Minutes

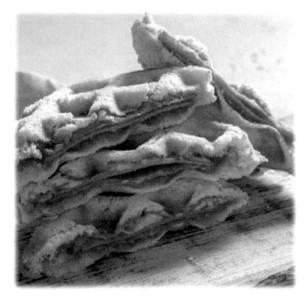

Ingredients:

✓ Cooking spray

✓ 2 Cervelat sausage, sliced into rounds

✓ 12 pieces pepperoni

Nutrition: **Calories**: 373; **Total Fat**: 24.4g

Saturated Fat: 6g; **Cholesterol**: 27mg

Sodium: 717mg; **Potassium**: 105mg

Total Carbohydrates: 28g; **Dietary Fiber**: 1.1g

Protein: 8.1g; **Total Sugars**: 4.5g

45. PIZZA FLAVORED CHAFFLE

❤ **Servings:** 2

🍰 **Preparation Time**: 6 Minutes

⏰ **Cooking Time**: 12 Minutes

Ingredients:

- ✓ 1 egg, beaten
- ✓ ½ cup cheddar cheese, shredded
- ✓ 2 tablespoons pepperoni, chopped
- ✓ 1 tablespoon keto marinara sauce
- ✓ 4 tablespoons almond flour
- ✓ 1 teaspoon baking powder
- ✓ ½ teaspoon dried Italian seasoning
- ✓ Parmesan cheese, grated

Directions:

1. Preheat your waffle maker.
2. In a bowl, mix the egg, cheddar cheese, pepperoni, marinara sauce, almond flour, baking powder, and Italian seasoning.
3. Add the mixture to the waffle maker.
4. Close the device and cook for some minutes.
5. Open it and transfer the chaffle to a plate.
6. Let cool for 2 minutes.
7. Repeat the steps with the remaining batter.
8. Top with the grated parmesan and serve.

Nutrition: **Calories**: 17; **Total Fat**: 14.3g

Saturated Fat: 7.5g; **Cholesterol**: 118mg

Sodium: 300mg; **Potassium**: 326mg

Total Carbohydrates: 1.8g; **Dietary Fiber**: 0.1g

Protein: 11.1g; **Total Sugars**: 0.4g

46. MAPLE CHAFFLE

❤ **Servings:** 2

🍰 **Preparation Time**: 10 Minutes

⏰ **Cooking Time**: 15 Minutes

Ingredients:

- ✓ 1 egg, lightly beaten
- ✓ 2 egg whites
- ✓ 1/2 teaspoon maple extract
- ✓ 2 teaspoons Swerve

- ✓ 1/2 teaspoon baking powder, gluten-free

- ✓ 2 tablespoons almond milk

- ✓ 2 tablespoons coconut flour

Directions:

1. Preheat your waffle maker.

2. In a bowl, whisk egg whites until stiff peaks form.

3. Stir in maple extract, Swerve, baking powder, almond milk, coconut flour, and egg.

4. Spray waffle maker with cooking spray.

5. Introduce half batter in the hot waffle maker and cook for 3-minutes or until golden brown. Repeat with the remaining batter.

6. Serve and enjoy.

Nutrition: **Calories**: 122; **Fat**: 6.6

Carbohydrates: 9; **Sugar**: 1; **Protein**: 7

Cholesterol: 82mg

47. CREAMY CHAFFLES

♥ **Servings:** 2

Preparation Time: 8 Minutes

⏰ **Cooking Time**: 5 Minutes

Ingredients:

- ✓ 1 cup egg whites

- ✓ 1 cup cheddar cheese, shredded

- ✓ 2 oz. Cocoa powder.

- ✓ 1 Pinch salt

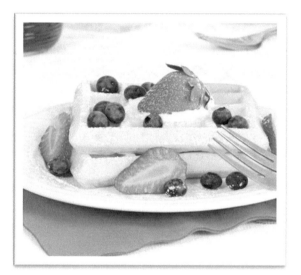

Topping:

- ✓ 4 oz. Cream cheese

- ✓ Strawberries

- ✓ Blueberries

- ✓ Coconut flour

Directions:

1. Beat the egg whites until fluffy and white

2. Chop Italian cheese with a knife and beat with egg whites.

3. Add cocoa powder and salt in the mixture and again beat.

4. Spray non-stick cooking spray into a round waffle maker.

5. Pour some batter into the waffle maker.

6. Cook the chaffle for about 5 minutes.

7. Once cooked, carefully remove the chaffle from the maker.

8. For serving, spread cream cheese on a chaffle. Top with strawberries, blueberries, and coconut flour.

9. Serve and enjoy!

Nutrition: **Protein:** 68; **Fat:** 187; **Carbohydrates**: 9

48. CHOCO AND SPINACH CHAFFLES

Servings: 2

Preparation Time: 10 Minutes

Cooking Time: 5 Minutes

Ingredients:

- ✓ 1 tablespoon. almond flour
- ✓ ½ cup chopped spinach
- ✓ 1/2 cup cheddar cheese
- ✓ 1 tablespoon cocoa powder
- ✓ ½ teaspoon baking powder
- ✓ 1 Large egg.
- ✓ 2 tablespoons Almond butter
- ✓ 1/2 teaspoon salt
- ✓ 1/2 teaspoon pepper

Directions:

1. Start by preheating the waffle iron

2. Blend all ingredients in a blender until mixed.

3. Pour 1/8 cup cheese into a waffle maker, and then pour the mixture into the greased waffle center.

4. Again, sprinkle cheese on the batter.

5. Cover.

6. Cook chaffles for about 4-5 minutes until cooked and crispy.

7. Once chaffles are cooked, remove and enjoy.

Nutrition: **Protein:** 4; **Fat:** 128; **Carbohydrates**: 11

49. PUMPKIN CHAFFLES WITH CHOCO CHIPS

♥ **Servings:** 2

Preparation Time: 6 Minutes

⏰ **Cooking Time**: 12 Minutes

Ingredients:

- ✓ 1 egg
- ✓ ½ cup shredded mozzarella cheese
- ✓ 4 teaspoons pureed pumpkin
- ✓ ¼ teaspoon pumpkin pie spice
- ✓ 2 tablespoons sweetener
- ✓ 1 tablespoon almond flour
- ✓ 4 teaspoons chocolate chips (sugar-free)

Directions:

1. Turn your waffle maker on.

2. In a bowl, beat the egg and stir in the pureed pumpkin.

3. Mix well.

4. Add the rest of the ingredients one by one.

5. Pour 1/3 of the mixture into your waffle maker.

6. Cook for 4 minutes.

7. Repeat the same steps with the remaining mixture.

Nutrition: **Calories**: 93; **Total Fat**: 7;

Saturated Fat: 3; **Cholesterol**: 69mg

Sodium: 13mg; **Potassium**: 48mg

Total Carbohydrates: 2; **Dietary Fiber**: 1

Protein: 7g; **Total Sugars**: 1g

50. RED VELVET CHAFFLE

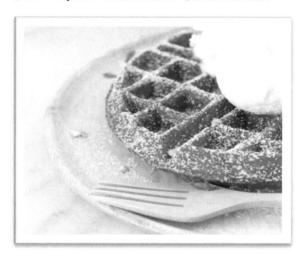

♥ **Servings:** 2

Preparation Time: 6 Minutes

⏰ **Cooking Time**: 12 Minutes

Ingredients:

- ✓ 1 egg
- ✓ ¼ cup mozzarella cheese, shredded
- ✓ 1 oz. Cream cheese
- ✓ 4 tablespoons almond flour
- ✓ 1 teaspoon baking powder
- ✓ 2 teaspoons sweetener
- ✓ 1 teaspoon red velvet extract
- ✓ 2 tablespoons cocoa powder

Directions:

1. Combine all the ingredients in a bowl.
2. Plug your waffle maker in.
3. Pour some batter into the waffle maker.
4. Seal and cook for four minutes.
5. Open and transfer to a plate.
6. Repeat the steps with the remaining batter.

Nutrition: **Calories**: 126; **Total Fat**: 10.1g

Saturated Fat: 3.4g; **Cholesterol**: 66mg

Sodium: 68mg; **Potassium**: 290mg

Total Carbohydrates: 6.5g; **Dietary Fiber**: 2.8g

Protein: 5.9g; **Total Sugars**: 0.2g

51. WALNUTS LOW CARB CHAFFLES

♥ **Servings:** 2

Preparation Time: 10 Minutes

Cooking Time: 5 Minutes

Ingredients:

- ✓ 2 tablespoons Cream cheese
- ✓ ½ teaspoon almonds flour
- ✓ ¼ teaspoon baking powder
- ✓ 1 Large egg
- ✓ ¼ cup chopped walnuts
- ✓ A pinch of stevia extract powder

Directions:

1. Preheat your waffle maker.
2. Spray the waffle maker with cooking spray.
3. In a bowl, add cream cheese, almond flour, baking powder, egg, walnuts, and Stevia.
4. Mix all ingredients.
5. Spoon the walnut batter in the waffle maker and cook for about 2-3 minutes.
6. Let chaffles cool at room temperature before serving.

Nutrition: **Protein**: 12%; **Fat**: 80%

Carbohydrates: 8%

52. CHAFFLE CREAM CAKE

♥ **Servings:** 2

🍫 **Preparation Time**: 10 Minutes

⏱ **Cooking Time**: 30Minutes

Ingredients: Chaffle:

- ✓ 4 oz. Cream cheese
- ✓ 4 eggs
- ✓ 1 tablespoon butter, melted
- ✓ 1 teaspoon vanilla extract
- ✓ ½ teaspoon cinnamon
- ✓ 1 tablespoon sweetener
- ✓ 4 tablespoons coconut flour
- ✓ 1 tablespoon almond flour
- ✓ 1 ½ teaspoons baking powder
- ✓ 1 tablespoon coconut flakes (sugar-free)
- ✓ 1 tablespoon walnuts, chopped

Frosting:

- ✓ 2 oz. Cream cheese
- ✓ 2 tablespoons butter
- ✓ 2 tablespoons sweetener
- ✓ ½ teaspoon vanilla

Directions:

1. Combine all the chaffle ingredients except coconut flakes and walnuts in a blender.

2. Blend until smooth.

3. Plug your waffle maker in.

4. Add some mixture to the waffle maker.

5. Cook for 3 minutes.

6. Repeat the steps until the remaining batter is used.

7. While letting the chaffles cool, make the frosting by combining all the ingredients.

8. Use a mixer to combine and turn frosting into a fluffy consistency.

9. Spread the frosting on top of the chaffles.

Nutrition: Calories: 127; **Total Fat:** 13.7g;

Saturated Fat: 9; **Cholesterol:** .9mg

Sodium: 107.3mg; **Potassium:** 457mg

Total Carbohydrates: 5.5g; **Dietary Fiber:** 1.3g

Protein: 5.3g; **Total Sugars:** 1.5g

53. SIMPLE PEANUT BUTTER CHAFFLE

💙 **Servings:** 2

🧇 **Preparation Time**: 5 Minutes

⏰ **Cooking Time**: 7-9 Minutes

Ingredients: For the Batter:

- ✓ 4 eggs
- ✓ 2 ounces cream cheese, softened
- ✓ ¼ cup creamy peanut butter
- ✓ 1 teaspoon vanilla extract
- ✓ 2 tablespoons stevia
- ✓ 5 tablespoons almond flour

Other:

- ✓ 1 tablespoon coconut oil to brush the waffle maker

Directions:

1. Preheat the waffle maker.

2. Add the eggs, cream cheese, and peanut butter to a bowl and stir with a wire whisk until combined.

3. Add the vanilla extract and Stevia and mix until combined.

4. Stir in the almond flour and stir until combined.

5. Brush the heated waffle maker with coconut oil and add a few tablespoons of the batter.

6. Cover and cook for about 7–8 minutes, depending on your waffle maker.

7. Serve and enjoy.

Nutrition: **Calories:** 291; **Fat:** 24.9g; **Carbs:** 5.9g; **Sugar:** 2; **Protein:** 12.5g; **Sodium:** 1mg

54. BEGINNER BROWNIES CHAFFLE

💙 **Servings:** 2

🧇 **Preparation Time**: 10 Minutes

⏰ **Cooking Time**: 5 Minutes

Ingredients:

- ✓ 1 cup cheddar cheese
- ✓ 1 tablespoon. cocoa powder
- ✓ ½ teaspoon baking powder
- ✓ 1 Large egg.
- ✓ ¼ cup melted keto chocolate chips for topping

Directions:

1. Preheat dash minutes waffle iron and grease it.

2. Blend all ingredients in a blender until mixed.

3. Pour one teaspoon of cheese into a waffle maker, and then pour the mixture in the center of the greased waffle.

4. Again, sprinkle cheese on the batter.

5. Cover.

6. Cook chaffles for about 4-5 minutes until cooked and crispy.

7. Once chaffles are cooked, remove them.

8. Top with melted chocolate, and enjoy!

Nutrition: **Protein**:7;   **Fat**:239;

Carbohydrates: 14

---

55. HOLIDAYS CHAFFLES

Servings: 2

Preparation Time: 5 Minutes

Cooking Time: 5 Minutes

Ingredients:

- ✓ 1 cup egg whites
- ✓ 2 teaspoons. Coconut flour
- ✓ ½ teaspoon Vanilla
- ✓ 1 teaspoon baking powder
- ✓ 1 teaspoon baking soda
- ✓ 1/8 teaspoon cinnamon powder
- ✓ 1 cup mozzarella cheese, grated

Topping:

- ✓ Cranberries
- ✓ Keto Chocolate sauce

Directions:

1. Make 4 minutes chaffles from the chaffle ingredients.

2. Top with chocolate sauce and cranberries

3. Serve hot and enjoy!

Nutrition: **Protein**:133;   **Fat**:201;

Carbohydrates: 18

---

56. BACON, EGG & AVOCADO CHAFFLE SANDWICH

♥ **Servings:** 2

🍞 **Preparation Time**: 10 Minutes

⏰ **Cooking Time**: 10 Minutes

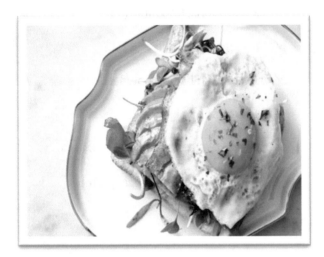

Ingredients:

- ✓ Cooking spray
- ✓ 4 Bacon Slices
- ✓ 2 eggs
- ✓ ½ Avocado, mashed
- ✓ 4 Basic chaffles
- ✓ 2 Lettuce leaves

Directions:

1. Coat your skillet with cooking spray.

2. Cook the bacon until golden and crisp.

3. Transfer into a paper towel-lined plate.

4. Break the eggs into the same pan and cook until firm.

5. Flip and cook until the yolk is set.

6. Spread the avocado on the chaffle.

7. Top with lettuce, egg, and bacon.

8. Top with another chaffle.

Nutrition: **Calories**: 372; **Total Fat**: 30.1g

Saturated Fat: 8.6g; **Cholesterol:** 205mg

Sodium: 3mg; **Total Carbohydrates:** 5.4g

Dietary Fiber: 3.4g; **Total Sugars:** 0.6g

Protein: 20.6g; **Potassium:** 524mg

57. SAUSAGE & EGG CHAFFLE SANDWICH

💜 **Servings:** 2

Preparation Time: 10 Minutes

⏰ **Cooking Time:** 10 Minutes

Ingredients:

- ✓ 2 Basic cooked chaffles
- ✓ 1 tablespoon olive oil
- ✓ 1 Sausage, sliced into rounds
- ✓ 1 egg

Directions:

1. Pour olive oil into your pan over medium heat.

2. Put it over medium heat.

3. Add the sausage and cook until brown on both sides.

4. Put the sausage rounds on top of one chaffle.

5. Cook the egg in the same pan without mixing.

6. Place on top of the sausage rounds.

7. Top with another chaffle.

Nutrition: Calories:332; TotalFat:21.6g; Saturated Fat: 4.4g; Cholesterol: 139mg; Potassium: 16g; Sodium: 463mg; Total Carbohydrates: 24.9g; Dietary Fiber: 0g; Protein: 10g; Total Sugars: 0.2g

58. BANANA NUT MUFFIN

💜 **Servings:** 2

Preparation Time: 6 Minutes

⏰ **Cooking Time:** 12 Minutes

Ingredients:

- ✓ 1 egg
- ✓ 1 oz. Cream cheese
- ✓ ¼ cup mozzarella cheese, shredded
- ✓ 1 teaspoon banana extract
- ✓ 2 tablespoons sweetener
- ✓ 1 teaspoon baking powder
- ✓ 4 tablespoons almond flour
- ✓ 2 tablespoons walnuts, chopped

Directions:

1. Combine all the ingredients in a bowl.

2. Turn on the waffle maker.

3. Add the batter to the waffle maker.

4. Seal and cook for four minutes.

5. Open and transfer the waffle to a plate. Let cool for two minutes.

6. Do the same steps with the remaining mixture.

Nutrition: Calories:169; TotalFat:14g; SaturatedFat:4.6g; Cholesterol:99mg; Sodium:98mg; Potassium:343mg; TotalCarbohydrates:5.6g; DietaryFiber: 2g; Protein: 5g; Total Sugars: 0.6g

59. CINNAMON ROLL CHAFFLES

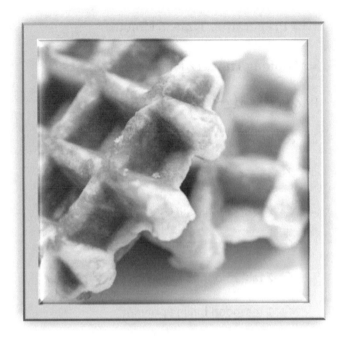

Directions:

1. Preheat the waffle maker and mix all ingredients in a bowl.

2. Pour the chaffle mixture into the center of the greased waffle maker.

3. Cover.

4. Cook chaffles for about 5 minutes until cooked and crispy.

5. Once chaffles are cooked, remove them.

6. Pour melted butter oil on top.

7. Serve and enjoy!

Nutrition: **Protein:** 47; **Fat:** 247; **Carbohydrates**: 9

♥ **Servings:** 2

Preparation Time: 10 Minutes

⏰ **Cooking Time**: 5 Minutes

Ingredients:

✓ 1 tablespoon almond flour

✓ 1 teaspoon cinnamon powder

✓ 1/2 cup cheddar cheese

✓ 1 tablespoon cocoa powder

✓ ½ teaspoon baking powder

✓ 1 Large egg.

✓ 2 tablespoons Peanut oil for topping

60. CHOCO CHIP LEMON CHAFFLE

♥ Servings: 2

🍪 Preparation Time: 10 Minutes

⏰ Cooking Time: 15 Minutes

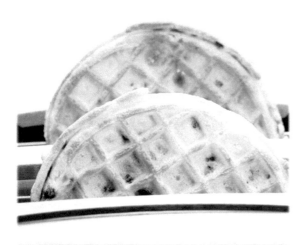

Ingredients:

- ✓ 2 eggs, lightly beaten
- ✓ 1 tablespoon unsweetened chocolate chips
- ✓ 2 teaspoons Swerve
- ✓ 1/2 teaspoon vanilla
- ✓ 1/2 teaspoon lemon extract
- ✓ 1/2 cup mozzarella cheese, shredded
- ✓ 2 teaspoons almond flour

Directions:

1. Preheat your waffle maker.

2. In a bowl, whisk eggs, Swerve, vanilla, lemon extract, cheese, and almond flour.

3. Add chocolate chips and stir well.

4. Spray waffle maker with cooking spray.

5. Pour 1/2 of the batter in the hot waffle maker and cook for 4-minutes or until golden brown. Repeat with the remaining batter.

6. Serve and enjoy.

Nutrition: **Calories:** 15; **Fat:** 10.8; **Carbohydrates:** 5.4; **Sugar:** 0.7; **Protein:** 9; **Cholesterol:** 167mg

61. CRUNCHY COCONUT CHAFFLES CAKE

♥ Servings: 2

🍪 Preparation Time: 5 Minutes

⏰ Cooking Time: 15 Minutes

Ingredients:

- ✓ 4 Large eggs
- ✓ 1 cup shredded cheese
- ✓ 2 tablespoons. Coconut cream
- ✓ 2 tablespoons. Coconut flour.

✓ 1 teaspoon stevia

For the Topping:

- ✓ 1 cup heavy cream
- ✓ 8 oz. Raspberries
- ✓ 4 oz. Blueberries
- ✓ 2 oz. Cherries

Directions:

1. Make four thin round chaffles with the chaffle ingredients. Once chaffles are cooked, set in layers on a plate.

2. Spread heavy cream to each layer evenly.

3. Top with raspberries, then blueberries and cherries.

4. Serve and enjoy!

> **Nutrition:** **Protein:** 67; **Fat:** 230; **Carbohydrates:** 21

62. COFFEE FLAVORED CHAFFLE

❤ **Servings:** 2

🥞 **Preparation Time:** 5 Minutes

⏰ **Cooking Time:** 7-9 Minutes

Ingredients: For the Batter:

- ✓ 4 eggs

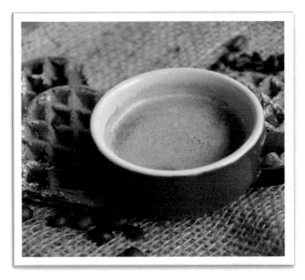

- ✓ 4 Ounces cream cheese
- ✓ ½ teaspoon vanilla extract
- ✓ 6 tablespoons strong boiled espresso
- ✓ ¼ cup stevia
- ✓ ½ cup almond flour
- ✓ 1 teaspoon baking powder
- ✓ A pinch of salt
- ✓ 2 tablespoons butter

Directions:

1. Preheat the waffle maker.

2. Add the eggs and cream cheese to a bowl and stir in the vanilla extract, espresso, Stevia, almond flour, baking powder, and salt pinch.

3. Stir just until everything is combined and fully incorporated.

4. Rub butter on the heated waffle maker

with butter and add a few tablespoons of the batter.

5. Cover and cook for about 7–8 minutes, depending on your waffle maker.

6. Serve and enjoy.

> **Nutrition:** **Calories:** 300; **Fat:** 26.g; **Carbs:** 4.8g; **Sugar:** 0.5; **Protein:** 10.8g; **Sodium:** 235mg

63. ITALIAN SAUSAGE CHAFFLES

🖤 **Servings:** 2

🧈 **Preparation Time:** 10 Minutes

⏲ **Cooking Time:** 8 Minutes

Ingredients:

- ✓ 1 egg, beaten
- ✓ 1 cup cheddar cheese, shredded
- ✓ ¼ cup Parmesan cheese, grated
- ✓ 1 lb. Italian sausage, crumbled
- ✓ 2 teaspoons baking powder
- ✓ 1 cup almond flour

Directions:

1. Preheat your waffle maker.

2. Mix all the ingredients in a bowl.

3. Introduce half of the mixture into the waffle maker.

4. Cover and cook for four minutes.

5. Transfer to a plate.

6. Let cool to make it crispy.

7. Do the same steps to make the next chaffle.

> **Nutrition:** **Calories:** 332; **Total Fat:** 27.1g
>
> **Saturated Fat:** 10.2g; **Cholesterol:** 9g
>
> **Sodium:** 634mg; **Total Carbohydrates:** 1.9g
>
> **Dietary Fiber:** 0.5g; **Total Sugars:** 0.1g
>
> **Protein:** 19.6g; **Potassium:** 359mg

64. CHAFFLES WITH STRAWBERRY FROSTY

🖤 **Servings:** 2

🧈 **Preparation Time:** 7 Minutes

⏲ **Cooking Time:** 5 Minutes

Ingredients:

- ✓ 1 cup frozen strawberries
- ✓ 1/2 cup Heavy cream
- ✓ 1 teaspoon stevia
- ✓ 1 Scoop protein powder
- ✓ 3 Keto chaffles

Directions:

1. Mix all ingredients in a mixing bowl.

2. Pour the mixture into silicone molds and freeze for about 4 hours to set.

3. Once the frosty is set, top on keto chaffles and enjoy!

Nutrition: **Protein**: 13%; **Fat**: 69%

Carbohydrates: 18%

Ingredients:

- ✓ 1 egg
- ✓ 2 tablespoons pecans, toasted and chopped
- ✓ 2 tablespoons almond flour
- ✓ 1 teaspoon erythritol
- ✓ 1/4 teaspoon pumpkin pie spice
- ✓ 1 tablespoon pumpkin puree
- ✓ 1/2 cup mozzarella cheese, grated

Directions:

1. Preheat your waffle maker.

2. Beat the egg in a small bowl.

3. Add remaining ingredients and mix well.

4. Spray the waffle maker with cooking spray.

5. Introduce half of the batter in the hot waffle maker and cook for four minutes or until golden brown. Repeat with the remaining batter.

6. Serve and enjoy.

Nutrition: **Calories**: 121; **Fat**:9g; **Carbohydrates**: 5.7; **Sugar**: 3.3; **Protein**: 6.7; **Cholesterol**: 86mg

---

65. PECAN PUMPKIN CHAFFLE

❤ **Servings**: 2

Preparation Time: 10 Minutes

Cooking Time: 15 Minutes

66. SWISS BACON CHAFFLE

💗 **Servings:** 2

🍰 **Preparation Time**: 10 Minutes

⏰ **Cooking Time**: 8 Minutes

Ingredients:

- ✓ 1 egg
- ✓ ½ cup Swiss cheese
- ✓ 2 tablespoons cooked crumbled bacon

Directions:

1. Preheat your waffle maker.
2. Beat the egg in a bowl.
3. Stir in the cheese and bacon.
4. Introduce half of the mixture into the device.
5. Close and cook for 4 minutes.
6. Cook the second chaffle using the same steps.

Nutrition: **Calories**: 23; **Total Fat**: 17.6g; **Saturated Fat**: 8.1g; **Cholesterol**: 128mg

Sodium: 522mg; **Total Carbohydrates**: 1.9g

Dietary Fiber: 0g; **Total Sugars**: 0.5g

Protein: 17.1g; **Potassium**: 158mg

67. BACON, OLIVES & CHEDDAR CHAFFLE

💗 **Servings:** 2

🍰 **Preparation Time**: 10 Minutes

⏰ **Cooking Time**: 8 Minutes

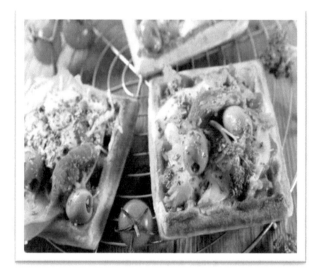

Ingredients:

- ✓ 1 egg
- ✓ ½ cup cheddar cheese, shredded
- ✓ 1 tablespoon black olives, chopped
- ✓ 1 tablespoon bacon bits

Directions:

1. Plug your waffle maker in.
2. In a bowl, beat the egg and stir in the cheese.
3. Add the black olives and bacon bits.
4. Mix well.

5. Add half of the mixture into the waffle maker.

6. Cover and cook for 4 minutes.

7. Open and transfer to a plate.

8. Let cool for 2 minutes.

9. Cook the other chaffle using the remaining batter.

Nutrition: **Calories**: 202; **Total Fat:** 16g

Saturated Fat: 8g; **Cholesterol**: 122mg; **Sodium**: 462mg; **Potassium**: 111mg; **Total Carbohydrates**: 0.9g; **Dietary Fiber**: 0.1g; **Protein**: 13.4g; **Total Sugars**: 0.3g

2. Beat the egg in a bowl.

3. Stir in the rest of the ingredients.

4. Introduce half of the batter into your waffle maker.

5. Cook for 4 minutes.

6. Remove the waffle and let sit for 2 minutes.

7. Do the same steps with the remaining batter.

Nutrition: **Calories**: 170; **Total Fat:** 14; **Saturated Fat**: 6; **Cholesterol**: 121mg; **Sodium**: 220mg; **Potassium**:165mg; **Total Carbohydrates**: 2; **Dietary Fiber**: 1; **Protein**: 10g; **Total Sugars**: 1g

68. GARLIC CHAFFLE

 Servings: 2

 Preparation Time: 10 Minutes

 Cooking Time: 8 Minutes

Ingredients:

- ✓ 1 egg
- ✓ ½ cup cheddar cheese, beaten
- ✓ 1 teaspoon coconut flour
- ✓ Pinch garlic powder

Directions:

1. Plug your waffle maker in.

69. HERBY CHAFFLE SNACKS

 Servings: 2

 Preparation Time: 8 Minutes

 Cooking Time: 28 Minutes

Ingredients:

- ✓ 1 egg, beaten
- ✓ ½ cup finely grated Monterey Jack cheese
- ✓ ¼ cup finely grated Parmesan cheese
- ✓ ½ teaspoon dried mixed herbs

Directions:

1. Preheat the waffle iron.

2. Add all ingredients to a medium bowl

3. Open the iron and pour in a quarter of the mixture. Close and cook until crispy, 7 minutes.

4. Remove the chaffle onto a plate and make three more with the rest of the ingredients.

5. Cut each chaffle into wedges and plate.

6. Allow cooling and serve.

Nutrition: Calories: 96; **Fats**: 6.29g; **Carbs**: 2.19g; **Net Carbs**: 2.19g; **Protein**: 42g

70. BREAKFAST SPINACH RICOTTA CHAFFLES

Servings: 2

Preparation Time: 8 Minutes

Cooking Time: 28 Minutes

Ingredients:

- ✓ 4 oz. Frozen spinach, thawed, squeezed dry
- ✓ 1 cup ricotta cheese
- ✓ 2 eggs, beaten
- ✓ ½ teaspoon garlic powder
- ✓ ¼ cup finely grated Pecorino Romano cheese
- ✓ ½ cup finely grated mozzarella cheese

- ✓ Salt
- ✓ Freshly ground black pepper to taste

Directions:

1. Preheat the waffle iron.

2. In a bowl, add all ingredients.

3. Open the iron, lightly grease with cooking spray, and spoon in a quarter of the mixture.

4. Close the iron and cook until brown and crispy, 7 minutes.

5. Remove the chaffle onto a plate and set it aside.

6. Make three more chaffles with the remaining mixture.

7. Allow cooling and serve afterward.

Nutrition: Calories: 1; **Fats**: 13.15g; **Carbs**: 5.06g; **Net Carbs**: 4.06g; **Protein**: 12.79g

71. PUMPKIN CHAFFLE WITH FROSTING

Servings: 2

Preparation Time: 10 Minutes

Cooking Time: 15 Minutes

Ingredients:

- ✓ 1 egg, lightly beaten

- ✓ 1 tablespoon sugar-free pumpkin puree
- ✓ 1/4 teaspoon pumpkin pie spice
- ✓ 1/2 cup mozzarella cheese, shredded

For the frosting:

- ✓ 1/2 teaspoon vanilla
- ✓ 2 tablespoons Swerve
- ✓ 2 tablespoons cream cheese, softened

Directions:

1. Preheat your waffle maker.

2. Add the egg to a bowl and whisk well.

3. Add pumpkin puree, pumpkin pie spice, and cheese and stir well.

4. Spray the waffle maker with cooking spray.

5. Pour 1/2 of the batter in the hot waffle maker and cook for 3-4 minutes or until golden brown. Repeat with the remaining batter.

6. In a small bowl, mix all frosting ingredients until smooth.

7. Add frosting on top of hot chaffles and serve.

Nutrition: **Calories**: 9.7; **Carbohydrates**: 3.6; **Sugar**: 0.6; **Protein**: 5.6; **Cholesterol**: 97mg

72. CHAFFLE STRAWBERRY SANDWICH

💔 **Servings:** 2

🧇 **Preparation Time**: 7 Minutes

⏰ **Cooking Time**: 5 Minutes

Ingredients:

- ✓ 1/4 cup heavy cream
- ✓ 4 oz. Strawberry slice

Chaffle Ingredients:

- ✓ 1 egg
- ✓ ½ cup mozzarella cheese

Directions:

1. Make two chaffles with the mentioned ingredients.

2. Meanwhile, mix cream and strawberries.

3. Spread this mixture over a chaffle slice.

4. Drizzle chocolate sauce over a sandwich.

5. Serve and enjoy!

Nutrition: **Protein**:4; **Fat**:196; **Carbohydrates**: 10

73. NEW YEAR KETO CHAFFLE CAKE

♥ **Servings:** 2

▨ **Preparation Time**: 0 Minutes

⏰ **Cooking Time**: 15 Minutes

Ingredients:

- ✓ 4 oz. Almond flour
- ✓ 2 cup cheddar cheese
- ✓ 5 eggs
- ✓ 1 teaspoon stevia
- ✓ 2 teaspoons baking powder
- ✓ 2 teaspoons vanilla extract
- ✓ 1/4 cup almond butter, melted
- ✓ 3 tablespoons Almond milk
- ✓ 1 cup cranberries
- ✓ I cup coconut cream

Directions:

1. Break the eggs into a small mixing bowl, mix the eggs, almond flour, Stevia, and baking powder.

2. Add the melted butter slowly to the flour mixture, mix well to ensure a smooth consistency.

3. Add the cheese, almond milk, cranberries, and vanilla to the flour and butter mixture; be sure to mix well.

4. Preheat the waffles maker and grease it with avocado oil.

5. Pour some mixture into the waffle maker and cook until golden brown.

6. Make five chaffles

7. Stag chaffles on a plate. Spread the cream all around.

8. Cut in slice and serve.

Nutrition:	Protein:15;	Fat:207;
Carbohydrates: 15		

Chapter 3. Sweets

74. CINNAMON SWIRL CHAFFLES

💔 **Servings**: 2

🍫 **Preparation Time**: 10 Minutes

⏱ **Cooking Time**: 12 Minutes

Ingredients: For the Chaffles:

- ✓ 1 Organic egg
- ✓ ½ cup Mozzarella cheese, shredded
- ✓ 1 tablespoon almond flour
- ✓ ¼ teaspoon organic baking powder
- ✓ 1 teaspoon granulated Erythritol
- ✓ 1 teaspoon ground cinnamon

For the Topping:

- ✓ 1 tablespoon butter
- ✓ 1 teaspoon ground cinnamon
- ✓ 2 teaspoons powdered Erythritol

Directions:

1. Preheat the waffle iron and then grease it.

2. For chaffles, place all ingredients and mix until well combined in a bowl.

3. For the topping, place all ingredients in a small microwave-safe bowl and microwave for about 15 seconds.

4. Remove from the microwave and mix well.

5. Place 1/3 of the chaffles mixture into the preheated waffle iron.

6. Top with 1/3 of the butter mixture, and with a skewer, gently swirl into the chaffles mixture.

7. Cook for about 3-4 minutes or until golden brown.

8. Repeat with the remaining chaffles and topping mixture.

9. Serve warm.

<u>Nutrition:</u> **Calories**: 87; **Net Carbs**: 1g; **Fat**: 7.4g; **Saturated Fat**: 3.5g; **Carbohydrates**: 2.1g

Dietary Fiber: 1.1g; **Sugar**: 0.2g; **Protein**: 3.3g

75. PROTEIN MOZZARELLA CHAFFLES

♥ **Servings:** 2

Preparation Time: 10 Minutes

🕐 **Cooking Time:** 20 Minutes

Ingredients:

- ✓ ½ Scoop unsweetened protein powder
- ✓ 2 Large organic eggs
- ✓ ½ cup Mozzarella cheese, shredded
- ✓ 1 tablespoon Erythritol
- ✓ ¼ teaspoon organic vanilla extract

Directions:

1. Get and preheat a mini waffle maker and then grease it.

2. In a medium bowl, place all ingredients, and with a fork, mix until well combined.

3. Place ¼ of the mixture into the preheated waffle iron and cook for about 4-5 minutes or until golden brown.

4. Repeat with the remaining mixture.

5. Serve warm.

Nutrition: Calories: 61; **Net Carbs:** 0.4g; **Fat:** 3.3g; **Saturated Fat:** 1.2g; **Carbohydrates:** 0.4g; **Dietary Fiber:** 0g; **Sugar:** 0.2g; **Protein:** 7.3g

76. MOZZARELLA & BUTTER CHAFFLES

♥ **Servings:** 2

Preparation Time: 10 Minutes

🕐 **Cooking Time:** 8 Minutes

Ingredients:

- ✓ 1 Large organic egg, beaten
- ✓ ¾ cup Mozzarella cheese, shredded
- ✓ ½ tablespoon unsalted butter, melted
- ✓ 2 tablespoons blanched almond flour
- ✓ 2 tablespoons Erythritol
- ✓ ½ teaspoon ground cinnamon
- ✓ ½ teaspoon Psyllium husk powder
- ✓ ¼ teaspoon organic baking powder
- ✓ ½ teaspoon organic vanilla extract

Directions:

1. Preheat a waffle maker and then grease it.

2. In a medium bowl, place all ingredients, and with a fork, mix until well combined.

3. Place half of the mixture into the preheated waffle iron and cook for about 3-5 minutes or until golden brown.

4. Repeat with the remaining mixture.

5. Serve warm.

Nutrition: **Calories:** 140; **NetCarbs:** 1.9g; **Fat:** 10.6g; **Saturated Fat:** 4g; **Carbohydrates:** 3g; **Dietary Fiber:** 1.1g **Sugar:** 0.3g; **Protein:** 7.8g

77. CREAM CHEESE CHAFFLES

♥ **Servings:** 2

▦ **Preparation Time:** 10 Minutes

⏰ **Cooking Time:** 8 Minutes

Ingredients:

- ✓ 2 teaspoons coconut flour
- ✓ 3 teaspoons Erythritol
- ✓ ¼ teaspoon organic baking powder
- ✓ 1 Organic egg, beaten
- ✓ 1 Ounce cream cheese, softened
- ✓ ½ teaspoon organic vanilla extract

Directions:

1. Preheat a mini waffle maker and then grease it.

2. In a bowl, place flour, Erythritol, and baking powder and mix well.

3. Add the egg, cream cheese, and vanilla extract and beat until well combined.

4. Place half of the mixture into the preheated waffle iron and cook for about 3-4 minutes or until golden brown.

5. Repeat with the remaining mixture.

6. Serve warm.

Nutrition: **Calories:** 95; **Net Carbs:** 1.6g; **Fat:** 7.4g; **Saturated Fat:** 4g; **Carbohydrates:** 2.6g **Dietary Fiber:** 1g; **Sugar:** 0.3g; **Protein:** 4.2g

78. CREAM CHEESE & BUTTER CHAFFLES

♥ **Servings:** 2

▦ **Preparation Time:** 10 Minutes

⏰ **Cooking Time:** 16 Minutes

Ingredients:

- ✓ 2 tablespoons butter, melted and cooled
- ✓ 2 Large organic eggs
- ✓ 2 ounces cream cheese, softened
- ✓ ¼ cup powdered Erythritol
- ✓ 1½ teaspoons organic vanilla extract
- ✓ A pinch of salt
- ✓ ¼ cup almond flour
- ✓ 2 tablespoons coconut flour
- ✓ 1 teaspoon organic baking powder

Directions:

1. Preheat a mini waffle maker and then grease it.

2. In a bowl, place the butter and eggs and beat until creamy.

3. Add the cream cheese, Erythritol, vanilla extract, and salt and beat until well combined.

4. Add the flour and baking powder and beat until well combined.

5. Place ¼ of the mixture into the preheated waffle iron and cook for about four minutes or until golden brown.

6. Repeat with the remaining mixture.

7. Serve warm.

Nutrition: **Calories**: 202; **Net Carbs**: 2.8g; **Fat**: 17.3g; **Saturated Fat**: 8g; **Carbohydrates**: 5.1g; **Dietary Fiber**: 2.3g; **Sugar**: 0.7g; **Protein**: 4.8g

Directions:

1. Preheat a mini waffle maker and then grease it.

2. In a medium bowl, place all ingredients, and with a fork, mix until well combined.

3. Place half of the mixture into the preheated waffle iron and cook for about 3-4 minutes or until golden brown.

4. Repeat with the remaining mixture.

5. Serve warm.

Nutrition: **Calories**: 112; **Net Carbs**: 1.6g

Fat: 6.9g; **Saturated Fat**: 2.7g; **Carbohydrates**: 3.7g; **Dietary Fiber**: 2.1g; **Sugar**: 0.2g; **Protein**: 10.9g

79. WHIPPING CREAM CHAFFLES

❤ **Servings:** 2

🧇 **Preparation Time**: 10 Minutes

⏰ **Cooking Time**: 8 Minutes

Ingredients:

- ✓ 1 Organic egg, beaten
- ✓ 1 tablespoon heavy whipping cream
- ✓ 2 tablespoons sugar-free peanut butter powder
- ✓ 2 tablespoons Erythritol
- ✓ ¼ teaspoon organic baking powder
- ✓ ¼ teaspoon peanut butter extract

80. ALMOND BUTTER CHAFFLES

❤ **Servings:** 2

🧇 **Preparation Time**: 5 Minutes

⏰ **Cooking Time**: 10 Minutes

Ingredients:

- ✓ 1 Large organic egg, beaten
- ✓ 1/3 cup Mozzarella cheese, shredded
- ✓ 1 tablespoon Erythritol
- ✓ 2 tablespoons almond butter
- ✓ 1 teaspoon organic vanilla extract

Directions:

1. Preheat a mini waffle maker and then grease it.

2. In a medium bowl, place all ingredients, and with a fork, mix until well combined.

3. Place half of the mixture into the preheated waffle iron and cook for about 3-5 minutes or until golden brown.

4. Repeat with the remaining mixture.

5. Serve warm.

Nutrition: **Calories**: 153; **Net Carbs**: 2g

Fat: 12.3g; **Saturated Fat**: 2g; **Carbohydrates**: 3.6g; **Dietary Fiber**: 1.6g; **Sugar**: 1.2g; **Protein**: 7.9g

81. PEANUT BUTTER CHAFFLES

♥ **Servings:** 2

▦ **Preparation Time**: 5 Minutes

⏰ **Cooking Time**: 8 Minutes

Ingredients:

- ✓ 1 Organic egg, beaten
- ✓ ½ cup Mozzarella cheese, shredded
- ✓ 3 tablespoons granulated Erythritol
- ✓ 2 tablespoons peanut butter

Directions:

1. Preheat a mini waffle maker and then grease it.

2. In a medium bowl, place all ingredients, and with a fork, mix until well combined.

3. Place half of the mixture into the preheated waffle iron and cook for about four minutes or until golden brown.

4. Repeat with the remaining mixture.

5. Serve warm.

Nutrition: **Calories**: 145; **Net Carbs**: 2.6g; **Fat**: 11.5g; **Saturated Fat**: 3.1g; **Carbohydrates**: 3.6g; **Dietary Fiber**: 1g; **Sugar**: 1.7g; **Protein**: 8.8g

82. LEMON CHAFFLES

♥ **Servings:** 2

Preparation Time: 10 Minutes

⏰ **Cooking Time**: 10 Minutes

Ingredients:

- ✓ 1 Organic egg, beaten
- ✓ 1 Ounce cream cheese, softened
- ✓ 2 tablespoons almond flour
- ✓ 1 tablespoon fresh lemon juice
- ✓ 2 teaspoons Erythritol
- ✓ ½ teaspoon fresh lemon zest, grated
- ✓ ¼ teaspoon organic baking powder
- ✓ A pinch of salt
- ✓ ½ teaspoon powdered Erythritol

Directions:

1. Preheat a mini waffle maker and then grease it.

2. In a bowl, place all ingredients except the powdered Erythritol and beat until well combined.

3. Place half of the mixture into the preheated waffle iron and cook for about 3-5 minutes or until golden brown.

4. Repeat with the remaining mixture.

5. Serve warm with the sprinkling of powdered Erythritol.

Nutrition: Calories:129; NetCarbs: 1.2g Fat: 10.9g; Saturated Fat: 4.1g; Carbohydrates: 2.4g; Dietary Fiber: 0.8g; Sugar: 0.6g; Protein: 3.9g

83. BLUEBERRY CHAFFLES

♥ **Servings:** 2

Preparation Time: 10 Minutes

⏰ **Cooking Time**: 20 Minutes

Ingredients:

- ✓ 1 cup Mozzarella cheese, shredded
- ✓ 2 tablespoons almond flour
- ✓ 1 teaspoon organic baking powder
- ✓ 2 Organic eggs
- ✓ 1 teaspoon ground cinnamon
- ✓ 1 tablespoon Erythritol
- ✓ 3 tablespoons fresh blueberries

Directions:

1. Preheat a mini waffle maker and then grease it.

2. In a bowl, place all ingredients except blueberries and beat until well combined.

3. Fold in the blueberries.

4. Place ¼ of the mixture into the preheated waffle iron and cook for about 3-5 minutes or until golden brown.

5. Repeat with the remaining mixture.

6. Serve warm.

Nutrition: Calories: 80; Net Carbs: 2.2g; Fat: 5.4g; Saturated Fat: 1.6g; Carbohydrates: 3.1g; Dietary Fiber: 0.9g; Sugar: 1g; Protein: 4.8g

84. BLUEBERRY CREAM CHEESE CHAFFLES

♥ **Servings:** 2

▦ **Preparation Time**: 10 Minutes

⏱ **Cooking Time**: 8 Minutes

Ingredients:

- ✓ 1 Organic egg, beaten
- ✓ 1 tablespoon cream cheese, softened
- ✓ 3 tablespoons almond flour
- ✓ ¼ teaspoon organic baking powder
- ✓ 1 teaspoon organic blueberry extract
- ✓ 5-6 Fresh blueberries

Directions:

1. Preheat a mini waffle maker and then grease it.

2. In a bowl, place all the ingredients except blueberries and beat until well combined.

3. Fold in the blueberries.

4. Divide the mixture into five portions.

5. Place one portion of the mixture into the preheated waffle iron and cook for about 3-4 minutes or until golden brown.

6. Repeat with the remaining mixture.

7. Serve warm.

Nutrition: **Calories:** 120; **Net Carbs:** 1.8g; **Fat:** 9.6g; **Saturated Fat:** 2.2g; **Carbohydrates:** 3.1g; **Dietary Fiber:** 1.3g; **Sugar:** 1g; **Protein:** 3.2g

85. BLACKBERRY CHAFFLES

♥ **Servings:** 2

▦ **Preparation Time**: 10 Minutes

⏱ **Cooking Time**: 8 Minutes

Ingredients:

- ✓ 1 Organic egg, beaten
- ✓ 1/3 cup Mozzarella cheese, shredded
- ✓ 1 teaspoon cream cheese, softened
- ✓ 1 teaspoon coconut flour
- ✓ ¼ teaspoon organic baking powder
- ✓ ¾ teaspoon powdered Erythritol
- ✓ ¼ teaspoon ground cinnamon
- ✓ ¼ teaspoon organic vanilla extract
- ✓ A pinch of salt
- ✓ 1 tablespoon fresh blackberries

Directions:

1. Preheat a mini waffle maker and then grease it.

2. In a bowl, place all the ingredients except for blackberries and beat until well combined.

3. Fold in the blackberries.

4. Place half of the mixture into the preheated waffle iron and cook for about four minutes or until golden brown.

5. Repeat with the remaining mixture.

6. Serve warm.

Nutrition: **Calories:** 121; **Net Carbs:** 2.7g; **Fat:** 7.5g; **Saturated Fat:** 3.3g; **Carbohydrates:** 4.5g; **Dietary Fiber:** 1.8g; **Sugar:** 0.9; **Protein:** 8.9g

86. STRAWBERRY CHAFFLES

❤ **Servings**: 2

🧇 **Preparation Time**: 10 Minutes

⏰ **Cooking Time**: 8 Minutes

Ingredients:

- ✓ 1 organic egg, beaten
- ✓ ¼ cup Mozzarella cheese, shredded
- ✓ 1 tablespoon cream cheese, softened
- ✓ ¼ teaspoon organic baking powder
- ✓ 1 teaspoon organic strawberry extract
- ✓ 2 fresh strawberries, hulled and sliced

Directions:

1. Preheat a mini waffle maker and then grease it.

2. In a bowl, place all ingredients except strawberry slices and beat until well combined.

3. Fold in the strawberry slices.

4. Place half of the mixture into the preheated waffle iron and cook for about four minutes or until golden brown.

5. Repeat with the remaining mixture.

6. Serve warm.

Nutrition: **Calories**: 69; **Net Carbs**: 1.6g; **Fat**: 4.6g; **Saturated Fat**: 2.2g; **Carbohydrates**: 1.9g; **Dietary Fiber**: 0.3g; **Sugar**: 1g; **Protein**: 4.2g

87. RASPBERRY CHAFFLES

❤ **Servings**: 2

🧇 **Preparation Time**: 10 Minutes

⏰ **Cooking Time**: 8 Minutes

Ingredients:

- ✓ 1 organic egg, beaten
- ✓ 1 tablespoon cream cheese, softened
- ✓ ½ cup Mozzarella cheese, shredded
- ✓ 1 tablespoon powdered Erythritol
- ✓ ¼ teaspoon organic raspberry extract
- ✓ ¼ teaspoon organic vanilla extract

Directions:

1. Preheat a mini waffle maker and then grease it.

2. In a medium bowl, place all ingredients, and with a fork, mix until well combined.

3. Place half of the mixture into the preheated waffle iron and cook for about four minutes or until golden brown.

4. Repeat with the remaining mixture.

5. Serve warm.

Nutrition: **Calories**: 69; **Net Carbs**: 0.6g; **Fat**: 5.2g; **Saturated Fat**: 2.5g; **Carbohydrates**: 0.6g; **Dietary Fiber**: 00g; **Sugar**: 0.2g; **Protein**: 5.6g

88. 2- BERRIES CHAFFLES

💝 **Servings**: 2

🧇 **Preparation Time**: 10 Minutes

⏰ **Cooking Time**: 10 Minutes

Ingredients:

- ✓ 1 organic egg
- ✓ 1 teaspoon organic vanilla extract
- ✓ 1 tablespoon of almond flour
- ✓ 1 teaspoon organic baking powder
- ✓ A pinch of ground cinnamon
- ✓ 1 cup Mozzarella cheese, shredded
- ✓ 2 tablespoons fresh blueberries
- ✓ 2 tablespoons fresh blackberries

Directions:

1. Preheat a waffle maker and then grease it.

2. In a bowl, place the egg and vanilla extract and beat well.

3. Add the flour, baking powder, and cinnamon and mix well.

4. Add the Mozzarella cheese and mix until just combined.

5. Gently fold in the berries.

6. Place half of the mixture into the preheated waffle iron and cook for about 4-5 minutes or until golden brown.

7. Repeat with the remaining mixture.

8. Serve warm.

Nutrition: **Calories**: 112; **Net Carbs**: 3.8g; **Fat**: 6.7g; **Saturated Fat**: 2.3g; **Carbohydrates**:

89. COCONUT & WALNUT CHAFFLES

💝 **Servings**: 2

🧇 **Preparation Time**: 10 Minutes

⏰ **Cooking Time**: 24 Minutes

Ingredients:

- ✓ 4 organic eggs, beaten
- ✓ 4 ounces cream cheese, softened
- ✓ 1 tablespoon butter, melted
- ✓ 4 tablespoons coconut flour
- ✓ 1 tablespoon almond flour
- ✓ 2 tablespoons Erythritol
- ✓ 1½ teaspoons organic baking powder
- ✓ 1 teaspoon organic vanilla extract
- ✓ ½ teaspoon ground cinnamon
- ✓ 1 tablespoon unsweetened coconut, shredded
- ✓ 1 tablespoon walnuts, chopped

Directions:

1. Preheat a mini waffle maker and then grease it.

2. In a blender, place all ingredients and pulse until creamy and smooth.

3. Divide the mixture into eight portions.

4. Place one portion of the mixture into the preheated waffle iron and cook for about 2-3 minutes or until golden brown.

5. Repeat with the remaining mixture.

6. Serve warm.

Nutrition: **Calories**: 125; **Net Carbs**: 2.2g

Fat: 10.2g; **Saturated Fat**: 5.2g; **Carbohydrates**: 4g; **Dietary Fiber**: 1.8g; **Sugar:** 0.4g; **Protein**: 4.6 g

90. CARROT CHAFFLES

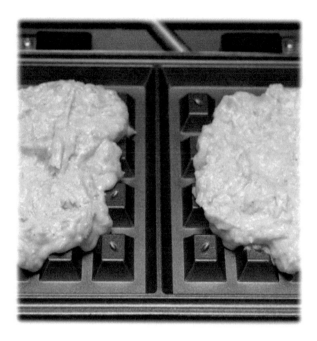

♥ **Servings**: 2

Preparation Time: 15 Minutes

⏰ **Cooking Time**: 18 Minutes

Ingredients:

- ✓ ¾ cup almond flour
- ✓ 1 tablespoon walnuts, chopped
- ✓ 2 tablespoons powdered Erythritol
- ✓ 1 teaspoon organic baking powder
- ✓ ½ teaspoon ground cinnamon
- ✓ ½ teaspoon pumpkin pie spice
- ✓ 1 Organic egg, beaten
- ✓ 2 tablespoons heavy whipping cream
- ✓ 2 tablespoons butter, melted
- ✓ ½ cup carrot, peeled and shredded

Directions:

1. Preheat a mini waffle maker and then grease it.

2. In a bowl, place the flour, walnut, Erythritol, cinnamon, baking powder, and spices and mix well.

3. Add the egg, heavy whipping cream, and butter, and mix until well combined.

4. Gently fold in the carrot.

5. Add about three tablespoons of the mixture into the preheated waffle iron and cook for about two and a half or three minutes or until golden brown.

6. Repeat with the remaining mixture.

7. Serve warm.

Nutrition: **Calories**: 165; **Net Carbs**: 2.4g

Fat: 14.7g; **Saturated Fat**: 4.4g; **Carbohydrates**: 4.4g; **Dietary Fiber**: 2g; **Sugar**: 1g; **Protein**: 1.5g

91. PUMPKIN CHAFFLES

Servings: 2

Preparation Time: 10 Minutes

Cooking Time: 12 Minutes

Ingredients:

✓ 1 Organic egg, beaten
✓ ½ cup Mozzarella cheese, shredded
✓ 1½ tablespoon homemade pumpkin puree
✓ ½ teaspoon Erythritol
✓ ½ teaspoon organic vanilla extract
✓ ¼ teaspoon pumpkin pie spice

Directions:

1. Preheat a mini waffle maker and then grease it.

2. In a bowl, place all the ingredients and beat until well combined.

3. Place ¼ of the mixture into the preheated waffle iron and cook for about 4-6 minutes or until golden brown.

4. Repeat with the remaining mixture.

5. Serve warm.

Nutrition: **Calories**: 59; **Net Carbs**: 1.2g; **Fat**: 3.5g; **Saturated Fat**: 1.5g; **Carbohydrates**: 1.6g; **Dietary Fiber**: 0.4g; **Sugar**: 0.7g; **Protein**: 4.9g

92. PUMPKIN & PSYLLIUM HUSK CHAFFLES

Nutrition: Calories: 46; Net Carbs: 0.6g

Fat: 2.8g; Saturated Fat: 1.1g; Carbohydrates: 0.8g; Dietary Fiber: 0.2g; Sugar: 0.4g; Protein:3.9g

Servings: 2

Preparation Time: 15 Minutes

Cooking Time: 18 Minutes

Ingredients:

- ✓ 2 Organic eggs
- ✓ ½ cup mozzarella cheese, shredded
- ✓ 1 tablespoon homemade pumpkin puree
- ✓ 2 teaspoons Erythritol
- ✓ ½ teaspoon psyllium husk powder
- ✓ 1/3 teaspoon ground cinnamon
- ✓ A pinch of salt
- ✓ ½ teaspoon organic vanilla extract

Directions:

1. Preheat a mini waffle maker and then grease it.

2. In a bowl, place all ingredients and beat until well combined.

3. Place ¼ of the mixture into the preheated waffle iron and cook for about 3-4 minutes or until golden brown.

4. Repeat with the remaining mixture.

5. Serve warm.

93. CINNAMON PUMPKIN CHAFFLES

♥ **Servings:** 2

▨ **Preparation Time:** 10 Minutes

⏰ **Cooking Time:** 16 Minutes

Ingredients:

- ✓ 2 Organic eggs
- ✓ 2/3 cup Mozzarella cheese, shredded
- ✓ 3 tablespoons sugar-free pumpkin puree
- ✓ 3 teaspoons almond flour
- ✓ 2 teaspoons granulated Erythritol
- ✓ 2 teaspoons ground cinnamon

Directions:

1. Preheat a mini waffle maker and then grease it.

2. In a medium bowl, place all ingredients, and with a fork, mix until well combined.

3. Place half of the mixture into the preheated waffle iron and cook for about four minutes or until golden brown.

4. Repeat with the remaining mixture.

5. Serve warm.

Nutrition: Calories: 63; Net Carbs: 1.4g Fat: 4g; Saturated Fat: 1.3g;Carbohydrates:2.5g Dietary Fiber: 1.1g; Sugar: 0.6g; Protein: 4.3g

94. SPICED PUMPKIN CHAFFLES

♥ **Servings:** 2

▨ **Preparation Time:** 10 Minutes

⏰ **Cooking Time:** 8 Minutes

Ingredients:

- ✓ 1 Organic egg, beaten
- ✓ ½ cup Mozzarella cheese, shredded
- ✓ 1 tablespoon sugar-free canned solid pumpkin
- ✓ ¼ teaspoon ground cinnamon
- ✓ A pinch of ground cloves
- ✓ A pinch of ground nutmeg
- ✓ A pinch of ground ginger

Directions:

1. Preheat a mini waffle maker and then grease it.

2. In a medium bowl, place all ingredients, and with a fork, mix until well combined.

3. Place half of the mixture into the preheated waffle iron and cook for about 3-4 minutes or until golden brown.

4. Repeat with the remaining mixture.

5. Serve warm.

Nutrition: Calories: 56; Net Carbs: 1g; Fat: 3.5g; Saturated Fat: 1.5g; Carbohydrates: 1.4g; Dietary Fiber: 0.4g; Sugar: 0.5g; Protein: 4.9g

95. WALNUT PUMPKIN CHAFFLES

Fat: 11.8g; Saturated Fat: 2g; Carbohydrates: 3.3g; Dietary Fiber: 1.7g; Sugar: 0.8g; Protein:6.7g

Servings: 2

Preparation Time: 10 Minutes

Cooking Time: 10 Minutes

Ingredients:

- ✓ 1 Organic egg, beaten
- ✓ ½ cup Mozzarella cheese, shredded
- ✓ 2 tablespoons almond flour
- ✓ 1 tablespoon sugar-free pumpkin puree
- ✓ 1 teaspoon Erythritol
- ✓ ¼ teaspoon ground cinnamon
- ✓ 2 tablespoons walnuts, toasted and chopped

Directions:

1. Preheat a mini waffle maker and then grease it.

2. In a bowl, place all ingredients except walnuts and beat until well combined.

3. Fold in the walnuts.

4. Place half of the mixture into the preheated waffle iron and cook for about 5 minutes or until golden brown.

5. Repeat with the remaining mixture.

6. Serve warm.

Nutrition: **Calories:** 148; **Net Carbs:** 1.6g

96. PUMPKIN CREAM CHEESE CHAFFLES

Servings: 2

Preparation Time: 10 Minutes

Cooking Time: 10 Minutes

Ingredients:

- ✓ 1 Organic egg, beaten
- ✓ ½ cup Mozzarella cheese, shredded
- ✓ 1½ tablespoon sugar-free pumpkin puree
- ✓ 2 teaspoons heavy cream
- ✓ 1 teaspoon cream cheese, softened
- ✓ 1 tablespoon almond flour
- ✓ 1 tablespoon Erythritol
- ✓ ½ teaspoon pumpkin pie spice
- ✓ ½ teaspoon organic baking powder
- ✓ 1 teaspoon organic vanilla extract

Directions:

1. Preheat a mini waffle maker and then grease it.

2. In a medium bowl, place all ingredients, and with a fork, mix until well combined.

3. Place half of the mixture into the preheated waffle iron and cook for about 3-5 minutes or until golden brown.

4. Repeat with the remaining mixture.

5. Serve warm.

> **Nutrition:** **Calories**: 110; **NetCarbs**:2.5g; **Fat:** 4.3g; **Saturated Fat**: 1g; **Carbohydrates**: 3.3g; **Dietary Fiber**: 0.8g; **Sugar:** 1g; **Protein**: 5.2g

97. WHIPPING CREAM PUMPKIN CHAFFLES

💜 **Servings:** 2

🧇 **Preparation Time**: 10 Minutes

⏰ **Cooking Time**: 12 Minutes

Ingredients:

- ✓ 2 Organic eggs
- ✓ 2 tablespoons homemade pumpkin puree
- ✓ 2 tablespoons heavy whipping cream
- ✓ 1 tablespoon coconut flour
- ✓ 1 tablespoon Erythritol
- ✓ 1 teaspoon pumpkin pie spice
- ✓ ½ teaspoon organic baking powder
- ✓ ½ teaspoon organic vanilla extract
- ✓ A pinch of salt
- ✓ ½ cup Mozzarella cheese, shredded

Directions:

1. Preheat a mini waffle maker and then grease it.

2. In a bowl, place all the ingredients except Mozzarella cheese and beat until well combined.

3. Add the Mozzarella cheese and stir to combine.

4. Place half of the mixture into the preheated waffle iron and cook for about 4-6 minutes or until golden brown.

5. Repeat with the remaining mixture.

6. Serve warm.

> **Nutrition:** **Calories**: 81; **Net Carbs**: 2.1g; **Fat:** 5.9g; **Saturated Fat**: 3g; **Carbohydrates**: 3.1g; **Dietary Fiber**: 1g; **Sugar**: 0.5g; **Protein**:4.3g

98. CHOCOLATE CREAM CHAFFLES

Nutrition: Calories: 76; Net Carbs: 2.1g; Fat: 5.9g; Saturated Fat: 3g; Carbohydrates: 3.8g; Dietary Fiber: 1.7g; Sugar: 0.3g; Protein: 3.8g

♥ **Servings:** 2

▦ **Preparation Time**: 10 Minutes

⏰ **Cooking Time**: 10 Minutes

Ingredients:

- ✓ 1 Organic egg
- ✓ 1½ tablespoons cacao powder
- ✓ 2 tablespoons Erythritol
- ✓ 1 tablespoon heavy cream
- ✓ 1 teaspoon coconut flour
- ✓ ½ teaspoon organic baking powder
- ✓ ½ teaspoon organic vanilla extract
- ✓ ½ teaspoon powdered Erythritol

Directions:

1. Preheat a mini waffle maker and then grease it.

2. In a bowl, place all ingredients except the powdered Erythritol and beat until well combined.

3. Place half of the mixture into the preheated waffle iron and cook for about 3-5 minutes or until golden brown.

4. Repeat with the remaining mixture.

5. Serve warm with the sprinkling of powdered Erythritol.

99. CHOCOLATE WHIPPING CREAM CHAFFLES

♥ **Servings:** 2

▦ **Preparation Time**: 10 Minutes

⏰ **Cooking Time**: 8 Minutes

Ingredients:

- ✓ 1 tablespoon almond flour
- ✓ 2 tablespoons cacao powder
- ✓ 2 tablespoons granulated Erythritol
- ✓ ¼ teaspoon organic baking powder
- ✓ 1 Organic egg
- ✓ 1 tablespoon heavy whipping cream
- ✓ ¼ teaspoon organic vanilla extract
- ✓ 1/8 teaspoon organic almond extract

Directions:

1. Preheat a mini waffle maker and then grease it.

2. In a bowl, place all ingredients and beat until well combined.

3. Place half of the mixture into the preheated waffle iron and cook for about four minutes or until golden brown.

4. Repeat with the remaining mixture.

5. Serve warm.

> **Nutrition:** **Calories:** 94; **Net Carbs**: 2g; **Fat:** 7.9g
>
> **Saturated Fat**: 3.2g; **Carbohydrates**: 3.9g
>
> **Dietary Fiber**: 1.9g; **Sugar**: 0.4g; **Protein**: 3.9g

Ingredients:

- ✓ 1 Large organic egg, beaten
- ✓ 1 Ounce cream cheese, softened
- ✓ 1 tablespoon sugar-free chocolate syrup
- ✓ 1 tablespoon Erythritol
- ✓ ½ tablespoon cacao powder
- ✓ ¼ teaspoon organic baking powder
- ✓ ½ teaspoon organic vanilla extract

Directions:

1. Preheat a mini waffle maker and then grease it.

2. In a medium bowl, place all ingredients, and with a fork, mix until well combined.

3. Place half of the mixture into the preheated waffle iron and cook for about 3-4 minutes or until golden brown.

4. Repeat with the remaining mixture.

5. Serve warm.

> **Nutrition:** **Calories:** 103; **Net Carbs**: 4.2g
>
> **Fat:** 7.7g; **Saturated Fat**: 4.1g; **Carbohydrates**: 4.6g; **Dietary Fiber**: 0.4g; **Sugar**: 2g; **Protein**: 4.5g

100. CHOCOLATE CREAM CHEESE CHAFFLES

💙 **Servings:** 2

🧱 **Preparation Time**: 10 Minutes

⏰ **Cooking Time**: 8 Minutes

Chapter 4. Savory

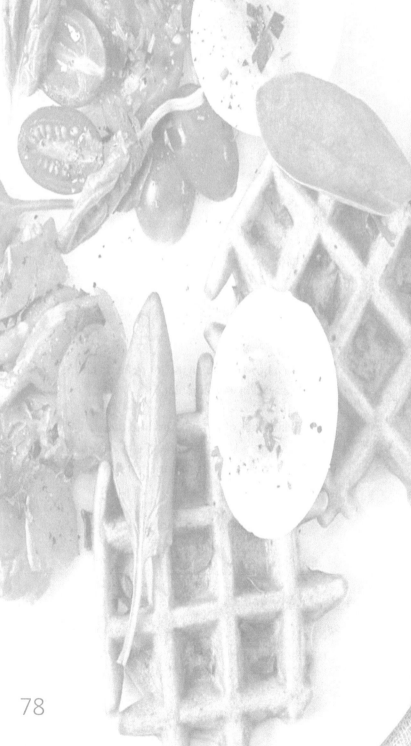

Nutrition: **Calories**: 150; **Net Carbs**: 0.6g; **Fat**: 11.9g; **Saturated Fat**: 6.7g; **Carbohydrates**: 0.6g; **Dietary Fiber**: 0g; **Sugar**: 0.3g; **Protein**: 10.2g

101. SIMPLE SAVORY CHAFFLES

❤ **Servings:** 2

🍫 **Preparation Time**: 5 Minutes

⏰ **Cooking Time**: 8 Minutes

Ingredients:

- ✓ 1 Large organic egg, beaten
- ✓ ½ cup Cheddar cheese, shredded
- ✓ A pinch of salt and freshly ground black pepper

Directions:

1. Preheat a mini waffle maker and then grease it.

2. In a bowl, place all the ingredients and beat until well combined.

3. Place half of the mixture into the preheated waffle iron and cook for about 3-4 minutes or until golden brown.

4. Repeat with the remaining mixture.

5. Serve warm.

78

102. GARLIC POWDER CHAFFLES

♥ **Servings:** 2

▦ **Preparation Time**: 5 Minutes

⏰ **Cooking Time**: 8 Minutes

Ingredients:

- ✓ 1 Organic egg, beaten
- ✓ ½ cup Monterrey Jack cheese, shredded
- ✓ 1 teaspoon coconut flour
- ✓ A pinch of garlic powder

Directions:

1. Preheat a mini waffle maker and then grease it.

2. In a bowl, place all the ingredients and beat until well combined.

3. Place half of the mixture into the preheated waffle iron and cook for about 3-4 minutes or until golden brown.

4. Repeat with the remaining mixture.

5. Serve warm.

Nutrition: Calories:147; NetCarbs:1.6g; Fat: 11.3g; Saturated Fat: 6.8g; Carbohydrates: 2.1g; Dietary Fiber: 0.5g; Sugar: 0.2g; Protein: 9g

103. GARLIC & ONION POWDER CHAFFLES

♥ **Servings:** 1

▦ **Preparation Time**: 5 Minutes

⏰ **Cooking Time**: 5 Minutes

Ingredients:

- ✓ 1 Organic egg, beaten
- ✓ ¼ cup Cheddar cheese, shredded
- ✓ 2 tablespoons almond flour
- ✓ ½ teaspoon organic baking powder
- ✓ ¼ teaspoon garlic powder
- ✓ ¼ teaspoon onion powder
- ✓ A pinch of salt

Directions:

1. Preheat a waffle iron and then grease it.

2. In a bowl, place all the ingredients and beat until well combined.

3. Place the mixture into the preheated waffle iron and cook for about 3-5 minutes or until golden brown.

4. Serve warm.

Nutrition: Calories: 274; Net Carbs: 3.3g; Fat: 21.3g; Saturated Fat: 7.8g; Carbohydrates: 5g; Dietary Fiber: 1.7g; Sugar: 1.4g; Protein: 12.8g

104. GARLIC POWDER & OREGANO CHAFFLES

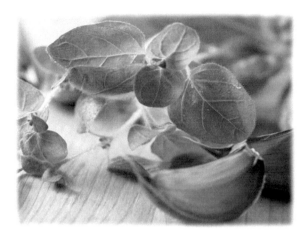

♥ **Servings:** 2

▦ **Preparation Time**: 5 Minutes

⏲ **Cooking Time**: 10 Minutes

Ingredients:

- ✓ ½ cup Mozzarella cheese, grated
- ✓ 1 Medium organic egg, beaten
- ✓ 2 tablespoons almond flour
- ✓ ½ teaspoon dried oregano, crushed
- ✓ ½ teaspoon garlic powder
- ✓ Salt, to taste

Directions:

1. Preheat a mini waffle maker and then grease it.

2. In a medium bowl, place all ingredients and mix until well combined.

3. Place half of the mixture into the preheated waffle iron and cook for about 4-5 minutes or until golden brown.

4. Repeat with the remaining mixture.

5. Serve warm.

> **Nutrition:** **Calories**: 100; **Net Carbs**: 1.4g; **Fat:** 7.2g; **Saturated Fat:** 1.7g; **Carbohydrates:** 2.4g; **Dietary Fiber**: 1g; **Sugar**: 0.6g; **Protein**: 4.9g

105. CHEDDAR PROTEIN CHAFFLES

♥ **Servings:** 2

▦ **Preparation Time**: 10 Minutes

⏲ **Cooking Time**: 40 Minutes

Ingredients:

- ✓ ½ cup golden flax seeds meal
- ✓ ½ cup almond flour
- ✓ 2 tablespoons unsweetened whey protein powder
- ✓ 1 teaspoon organic baking powder
- ✓ Salt and freshly ground black pepper, to taste

- ✓ ¾ cup Cheddar cheese, shredded
- ✓ 1/3 cup unsweetened almond milk
- ✓ 2 tablespoons unsalted butter, melted
- ✓ 2 large organic eggs, beaten

Directions:

1. Preheat a mini waffle maker and then grease it.

2. In a large bowl, place flax seeds meal, flour, protein powder, and baking powder and mix well.

3. Stir in the Cheddar cheese.

4. In another bowl, place the remaining ingredients and beat until well combined.

5. Add the egg mixture into the bowl with flax seeds meal mixture and mix until well combined.

6. Place the desired amount of the mixture into the preheated waffle iron and cook for about 4-5 minutes or until golden brown.

7. Repeat with the remaining mixture.

8. Serve warm.

Nutrition: Calories: 187; Net Carbs: 1.8g; Fat: 14.5g; Saturated Fat: 5g; Carbohydrates: 4.9g; Dietary Fiber: 3.1g; Sugar: 0.4g; Protein: 8g

106. SOUR CREAM PROTEIN CHAFFLES

♥ **Servings:** 2

Preparation Time: 10 Minutes

⏰ **Cooking Time**: 16 Minutes

Ingredients:

- ✓ 6 Organic eggs
- ✓ ½ cup sour cream
- ✓ ½ cup unsweetened whey protein powder
- ✓ 1 teaspoon organic baking powder
- ✓ ½ teaspoon salt
- ✓ 1 cup Cheddar cheese, shredded

Directions:

1. Preheat a waffle iron and then grease it.

2. In a medium bowl, place all ingredients and mix until well combined.

3. Place ¼ of the mixture into the preheated waffle iron and cook for about 3-4 minutes or until golden brown.

4. Repeat with the remaining mixture.

5. Serve warm.

Nutrition: Calories: 324; Net Carbs: 3.6g; Fat:22.6g; Saturated Fat: 11.9g; Carbohydrates: 3.6g; Dietary Fiber: 0g; Sugar: 1.3g; Protein: 27.3g

107. BASIL CHAFFLES

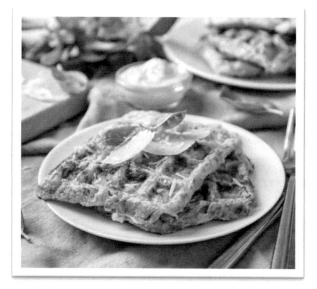

💜 **Servings:** 2

🧇 **Preparation Time**: 10 Minutes

⏰ **Cooking Time**: 16 Minutes

Ingredients:

- ✓ 2 Organic eggs, beaten
- ✓ ½ cup Mozzarella cheese, shredded
- ✓ 1 tablespoon Parmesan cheese, grated
- ✓ 1 teaspoon dried basil, crushed
- ✓ A pinch of salt

Directions:

1. Preheat a mini waffle maker and then grease it.
2. In a medium bowl, place all ingredients and mix until well combined.
3. Place 1/3 of the mixture into the preheated waffle iron and cook for about 3-4 minutes or until golden brown.
4. Repeat with the remaining mixture.
5. Serve warm.

> **Nutrition:** **Calories:** 61; **Net Carbs**: 0.4g;
> **Fat:** 4.2g
> **Saturated Fat**: 1.6g; **Carbohydrates**: 0.4g
> **Dietary Fiber**: 0g; **Sugar**: 0.2g; **Protein**: 5.7g

108. SAGE & COCONUT MILK CHAFFLES

💜 **Servings:** 2

🧇 **Preparation Time**: 10 Minutes

⏰ **Cooking Time**: 24 Minutes

Ingredients:

- ✓ ¾ cup coconut flour sifted
- ✓ 1½ teaspoons organic baking powder
- ✓ ½ teaspoon dried ground sage
- ✓ 1/8 teaspoon garlic powder
- ✓ 1/8 teaspoon salt
- ✓ 1 Organic egg

- ✓ 1 cup unsweetened coconut milk
- ✓ ¼ cup water
- ✓ 1½ tablespoons coconut oil, melted
- ✓ ½ cup cheddar cheese, shredded

Directions:

1. Preheat a waffle iron and then grease it.

2. In a bowl, add the flour, baking powder, sage, garlic powder, and salt and mix well.

3. Add the egg, coconut milk, water, and coconut oil and mix until a stiff mixture forms.

4. Add the cheese and gently stir to combine.

5. Divide the mixture into six portions.

6. Place one portion of the mixture into the preheated waffle iron and cook for about four minutes or until golden brown.

7. Repeat with the remaining mixture.

8. Serve warm.

Nutrition: **Calories**: 147; **Net Carbs**: 2.2g; **Fat**: 13g; **Saturated Fat**: 10.7g; **Carbohydrates**: 2.9g; **Dietary Fiber**: 0.7g; **Sugar**: 1.3g; **Protein**: 4g

109. DRIED HERBS CHAFFLES

♥ **Servings:** 2

🍳 **Preparation Time**: 5 Minutes

⏰ **Cooking Time**: 8 Minutes

Ingredients:

- ✓ 1 Organic egg, beaten
- ✓ ½ cup Cheddar cheese, shredded
- ✓ 1 tablespoon almond flour
- ✓ A pinch of dried thyme, crushed
- ✓ A pinch of dried rosemary, crushed

Directions:

1. Preheat a mini waffle maker and then grease it.

2. In a bowl, place all the ingredients and beat until well combined.

3. Place half of the mixture into the preheated waffle iron and cook for about 3-4 minutes or until golden brown.

4. Repeat with the remaining mixture.

5. Serve warm.

Nutrition: **Calories**: 168; **Net Carbs**: 0.9g; **Fat**: 13.4g; **Saturated Fat**: 6.8g; **Carbohydrates**: 1.3g; **Dietary Fiber**: 0.4g; **Sugar**: 0.4g; **Protein**: 9.8g

110. 3-CHEESES HERBED CHAFFLES

Servings: 2

Preparation Time: 10 Minutes

Cooking Time: 12 Minutes

Ingredients:

- ✓ 4 tablespoons almond flour
- ✓ 1 tablespoon coconut flour
- ✓ 1 teaspoon mixed dried herbs
- ✓ ½ teaspoon organic baking powder
- ✓ ¼ teaspoon garlic powder
- ✓ ¼ teaspoon onion powder
- ✓ Salt and freshly ground black pepper, to taste
- ✓ ¼ cup cream cheese softened
- ✓ 3 Large organic eggs
- ✓ ½ cup Cheddar cheese, grated
- ✓ 1/3 cup Parmesan cheese, grated

Directions:

1. Preheat a waffle iron and then grease it.

2. In a bowl, mix together the flours, dried herbs, baking powder, and seasoning and mix well.

3. In a separate bowl, put cream cheese and eggs and beat until well combined.

4. Add the flour mixture, cheddar, and Parmesan cheese and mix until well combined.

5. Place the desired amount of the mixture into the preheated waffle iron and cook for about 2-3 minutes or until golden brown.

6. Repeat with the remaining mixture.

7. Serve warm.

> **Nutrition:** **Calories**: 240; **Net Carbs**: 2.6g; **Fat**: 19g; **Saturated Fat**: 8.5g; **Carbohydrates**: 4g
>
> **Dietary Fiber**: 1.6g **Sugar**: 0.7g; **Protein**: 12.3g

111. ITALIAN SEASONING CHAFFLES

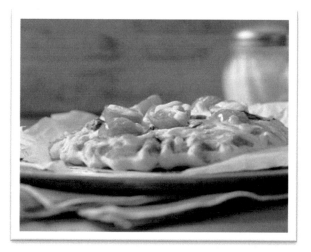

Servings: 2

Preparation Time: 10 Minutes

Cooking Time: 8 Minutes

Ingredients:

- ✓ ½ cup Mozzarella cheese, shredded
- ✓ 1 tablespoon Parmesan cheese, shredded
- ✓ 1 Organic egg
- ✓ ¾ teaspoon coconut flour
- ✓ ¼ teaspoon organic baking powder
- ✓ 1/8 teaspoon Italian seasoning
- ✓ A pinch of salt

Directions:

1. Preheat a mini waffle maker and then grease it.

2. In a medium bowl, place all ingredients, and with a fork, mix until well combined.

3. Place half of the mixture into the preheated waffle iron and cook for about 3-4 minutes or until golden brown.

4. Repeat with the remaining mixture.

5. Serve warm.

Nutrition: Calories: 86; **Net Carbs:** 1.9g; **Fat:** 5g; **Saturated Fat:** 2.6g; **Carbohydrates:** 3.8g **Dietary Fiber:** 1.9g; **Sugar:** 0.6g; **Protein:** 6.5g

112. GARLIC HERB BLEND SEASONING CHAFFLES

❤ **Servings:** 2

Preparation Time: 10 Minutes

⏰ **Cooking Time:** 8 Minutes

Ingredients:

- ✓ 1 Large organic egg, beaten
- ✓ ¼ cup Parmesan cheese, shredded
- ✓ ¼ cup Mozzarella cheese, shredded
- ✓ ½ tablespoon butter, melted
- ✓ 1 teaspoon garlic herb blend seasoning
- ✓ Salt, to taste

Directions:

1. Preheat a mini waffle maker and then grease it.

2. In a bowl, place all the ingredients and beat until well combined.

3. Place half of the mixture into the preheated waffle iron and cook for about 3-4 minutes or until golden brown.

4. Repeat with the remaining mixture.

5. Serve warm.

Nutrition: Calories: 115; **Net Carbs:** 1.1g; **Fat:** 8.8g; **Saturated Fat:** 4.7g; **Carbohydrates:** 1.2g; **Dietary Fiber:** 0.1g; **Sugar:** 0.2g; **Protein:** 8g

113. BBQ RUB CHAFFLES

💗 **Servings**: 2

🍰 **Preparation Time**: 5 Minutes

⏰ **Cooking Time**: 20 Minutes

Ingredients:

- ✓ 2 Organic eggs, beaten
- ✓ 1 cup Cheddar cheese, shredded
- ✓ ½ teaspoon BBQ rub
- ✓ ¼ teaspoon organic baking powder

Directions:

1. Preheat a mini waffle maker and then grease it.

2. In a medium bowl, place all ingredients, and with a fork, mix until well combined.

3. Place ¼ of the mixture into the preheated waffle iron and cook for about 5 minutes or until golden brown.

4. Repeat with the remaining mixture.

5. Serve warm.

Nutrition: **Calories**: 146; **Net Carbs**: 0.7g; **Fat**: 11.6g; **Saturated Fat**: 6.6g; **Carbohydrates**: 0.7g; **Dietary Fiber**: 0g; **Sugar**: 0.3g; **Protein**: 9.8g

114. BAGEL SEASONING CHAFFLES

💗 **Servings**: 2

🍰 **Preparation Time**: 10 Minutes

⏰ **Cooking Time**: 20 Minutes

Ingredients:

- ✓ 1 Large organic egg
- ✓ 1 cup Mozzarella cheese, shredded
- ✓ 1 tablespoon almond flour
- ✓ 1 teaspoon organic baking powder
- ✓ 2 teaspoons bagel seasoning
- ✓ ¼ teaspoon garlic powder
- ✓ ¼ teaspoon onion powder

Directions:

1. Preheat a mini waffle maker and then grease it.

2. In a medium bowl, place all ingredients, and with a fork, mix until well combined.

3. Place ¼ of the mixture into the preheated waffle iron and cook for about 3-4 minutes or until golden brown.

4. Repeat with the remaining mixture.

5. Serve warm.

Nutrition: **Calories**: 73; **Net Carbs**: 2g; **Fat**: 5.5g; **Saturated Fat**: 1.5g; **Carbohydrates**: 2.3g

Dietary Fiber: 0.3g; **Sugar**: 0.9g; **Protein**: 3.7g

115. ROSEMARY CHAFFLES

♥ **Servings**: 2

🍰 **Preparation Time**: 5 Minutes

⏱ **Cooking Time**: 8 Minutes

Ingredients:

- ✓ 1 Organic egg, beaten
- ✓ ½ cup Cheddar cheese, shredded
- ✓ 1 tablespoon almond flour
- ✓ 1 tablespoon fresh rosemary, chopped
- ✓ A pinch of salt and freshly ground black pepper

Directions:

1. Preheat a mini waffle maker and then grease it.

2. For the chaffles, in a medium bowl, place all ingredients and with a fork, mix until well combined.

3. Place half of the mixture into the preheated waffle iron and cook for about 3-4 minutes or until golden brown.

4. Repeat with the remaining mixture.

5. Serve warm.

Nutrition: **Calories**: 173; **Net Carbs**: 1.1g; **Fat**: 13.7g; **Saturated Fat**: 6.9g; **Carbohydrates**: 2.2g; **Dietary Fiber**: 1.1g; **Sugar**: 0.4g; **Protein**: 9.9g

116. LEMONY FRESH HERBS CHAFFLES

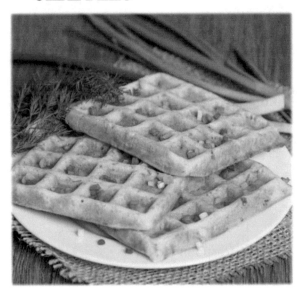

♥ **Servings**: 2

🍰 **Preparation Time**: 15 Minutes

⏱ **Cooking Time**: 24 Minutes

Ingredients:

- ✓ ½ cup ground flaxseed
- ✓ 2 Organic eggs
- ✓ ½ cup goat cheddar cheese, grated
- ✓ 2-4 tablespoons plain Greek yogurt
- ✓ 1 tablespoon avocado oil
- ✓ ½ teaspoon baking soda
- ✓ 1 teaspoon fresh lemon juice
- ✓ 2 tablespoons fresh chives, minced
- ✓ 1 tablespoon fresh basil, minced
- ✓ ½ tablespoon fresh mint, minced
- ✓ ¼ tablespoon fresh thyme, minced
- ✓ ¼ tablespoon fresh oregano, minced
- ✓ Salt and freshly ground black pepper, to taste

Directions:

1. Preheat a waffle iron and then grease it.

2. In a medium bowl, place all ingredients, and with a fork, mix until well combined.

3. Divide the mixture into six portions.

4. Place one portion of the mixture into the preheated waffle iron and cook for about four minutes or until golden brown.

5. Repeat with the remaining mixture.

6. Serve warm.

Nutrition: **Calories**: 117; **Net Carbs**: 0.9g; **Fat**: 7.9g; **Saturated Fat**: 3g; **Carbohydrates**: 3.7g; **Dietary Fiber**: 2.8g; **Sugar**: 0.7g; **Protein**: 6.4g

117. SCALLION CHAFFLES

Servings: 2

Preparation Time: 10 Minutes

Cooking Time: 8 Minutes

Ingredients:

- ✓ 1 Organic egg, beaten
- ✓ ½ cup Mozzarella cheese, shredded
- ✓ 1 tablespoon scallion, chopped
- ✓ ½ teaspoon Italian seasoning

Directions:

1. Preheat a mini waffle maker and then grease it.

2. In a medium bowl, place all ingredients, and with a fork, mix until well combined.

3. Place half of the mixture into the preheated waffle iron and cook for about four minutes or until golden brown.

4. Repeat with the remaining mixture.

5. Serve warm.

Nutrition: **Calories**: 56; **Net Carbs**: 0.7g; **Fat**: 3.8g; **Saturated Fat**: 1.5g; **Carbohydrates**: 0.8g; **Dietary Fiber**: 0.g; **Sugar**: 0.3g; **Protein**: 4.8g

118. JALAPEÑO CHAFFLES

♥ **Servings:** 2

▨ **Preparation Time**: 5 Minutes

⏱ **Cooking Time**: 10 Minutes

Ingredients:

- ✓ 1 Organic egg, beaten
- ✓ ½ cup Cheddar cheese, shredded
- ✓ ½ tablespoon jalapeño pepper, chopped
- ✓ Salt, to taste

Directions:

1. Preheat a mini waffle maker and then grease it.

2. In a medium bowl, place all ingredients, and with a fork, mix until well combined.

3. Place half of the mixture into the preheated waffle iron and cook for about 3-5 minutes or until golden brown.

4. Repeat with the remaining mixture.

5. Serve warm.

Nutrition: **Calories**: 146; **Net Carbs**: 0.6g; **Fat**: 11.6g; **Saturated Fat**: 6.6g; **Carbohydrates**: 0.6g; **Dietary Fiber**: 0g; **Sugar**: 0.4g; **Protein**: 9.8g

119. HOT SAUCE JALAPEÑO CHAFFLES

♥ **Servings:** 2

▨ **Preparation Time**: 10 Minutes

⏱ **Cooking Time**: 8 Minutes

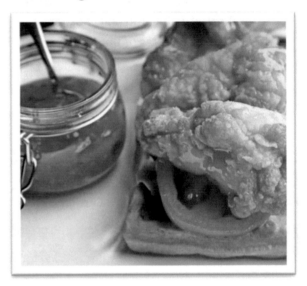

Ingredients:

- ✓ ½ cup plus 2 teaspoons Cheddar cheese, shredded and divided
- ✓ 1 Organic egg, beaten
- ✓ 6 Jalapeño pepper slices
- ✓ ¼ teaspoon hot sauce
- ✓ A pinch of salt

Directions:

1. Preheat a mini waffle maker and then grease it.

2. In a bowl, place ½ cup of cheese and the

remaining ingredients and mix until well combined.

3. Place about one teaspoon of cheese in the bottom of the waffle maker for about 30 seconds before adding the mixture.

4. Place half of the mixture into the preheated waffle iron and cook for about 3-4 minutes or until golden brown.

5. Repeat with the remaining cheese and mixture.

6. Serve warm.

Nutrition: **Calories**: 153; **Net Carbs**: 0.6g; **Fat**: 12.2g; **Saturated Fat**: 7g; **Carbohydrates**: 0.7g; **Dietary Fiber**: 0.1g; **Sugar**: 0.4g; **Protein**: 10.3g

120. SPINACH CHAFFLES

Servings: 2

Preparation Time: 10 Minutes

Cooking Time: 20 Minutes

Ingredients:

- ✓ 1 large organic egg, beaten
- ✓ 1 cup ricotta cheese, crumbled
- ✓ ½ cup Mozzarella cheese, shredded
- ✓ ¼ cup Parmesan cheese, grated
- ✓ 4 ounces frozen spinach, thawed and squeezed
- ✓ 1 garlic clove, minced
- ✓ Salt and freshly ground black pepper, to taste

Directions:

1. Preheat a mini waffle maker and then grease it.

2. In a medium bowl, place all ingredients and mix until well combined.

3. Place ¼ of the mixture into the preheated waffle iron and cook for about 4-5 minutes or until golden brown.

4. Repeat with the remaining mixture.

5. Serve warm.

Nutrition: **Calories**: 139; **Net Carbs**: 4.3g; **Fat**: 8.1g; **Saturated Fat**: 4g; **Carbohydrates**: 4.7g; **Dietary Fiber**: 0.4g; **Sugar**: 0.4g; **Protein**: 12.5g

121. CAULIFLOWER & CHIVES CHAFFLES

Nutrition: **Calories:** 107; **Net Carbs:** 1.2g; **Fat:** 7.3g; **Saturated Fat:** 4g; **Carbohydrates:** 1.7g

Dietary Fiber: 0.5g; **Sugar:** 0.7g; **Protein:** 8.8g

❤️ **Servings:** 2

Preparation Time: 10 Minutes

⏱️ **Cooking Time:** 48 Minutes

Ingredients:

- ✓ 1½ cups cauliflower, grated
- ✓ ½ cup Cheddar cheese, shredded
- ✓ ½ cup Mozzarella cheese, shredded
- ✓ ¼ cup Parmesan cheese, shredded
- ✓ 3 large organic eggs, beaten
- ✓ 3 tablespoons fresh chives, chopped
- ✓ ¼ teaspoon red pepper flakes, crushed
- ✓ Salt and freshly ground black pepper, to taste

Directions:

1. Preheat a mini waffle maker and then grease it.

2. In a food processor, Place all the ingredients and pulse until well combined.

3. Divide the mixture into eight portions.

4. Place one portion of the mixture into the preheated waffle iron and cook for about 5-6 minutes or until golden brown.

5. Repeat with the remaining mixture.

6. Serve warm.

122. CAULIFLOWER & ITALIAN SEASONING CHAFFLES

❤️ **Servings:** 2

Preparation Time: 10 Minutes

⏱️ **Cooking Time:** 20 Minutes

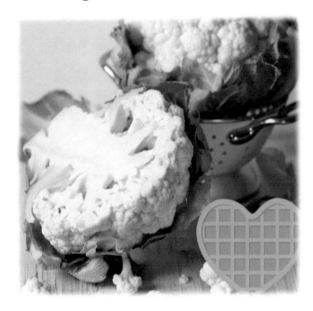

Ingredients:

- ✓ 1 cup cauliflower rice
- ✓ ¼ teaspoon garlic powder
- ✓ ½ teaspoon Italian seasoning
- ✓ Salt and freshly ground black pepper, to taste
- ✓ ½ cup Mexican blend cheese, shredded
- ✓ 1 Organic egg, beaten
- ✓ ½ cup Parmesan cheese, shredded

Directions:

1. Preheat a mini waffle maker and then grease it.

2. In a blender, add all the ingredients except Parmesan cheese and pulse until well combined.

3. Place 1½ tablespoon of the Parmesan cheese in the bottom of the preheated waffle iron.

4. Place ¼ of the egg mixture over the cheese and sprinkle with the ½ tablespoon of the Parmesan cheese.

5. Cook for about 4-5 minutes or until golden brown.

6. Repeat with the remaining mixture and Parmesan cheese.

7. Serve warm.

Nutrition:Calories:127;**NetCarbs**:2g;**Fat**:9g ;**SaturatedFat**:5.3g;**Carbohydrates**:2.7g;**Dietary Fiber**: 0.7g;**Sugar**:1.5g;**Protein**: 9.2g

123. ZUCCHINI & ONION CHAFFLES

Servings: 2

Preparation Time: 10 Minutes

Cooking Time: 16 Minutes

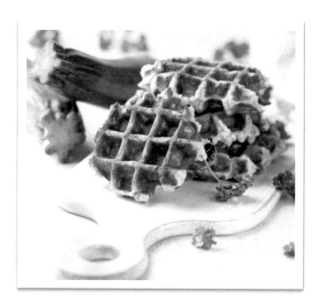

Ingredients:

- ✓ 2 cups zucchini, grated and squeezed
- ✓ ½ cup onion, grated and squeezed
- ✓ 2 Organic eggs
- ✓ ½ cup Mozzarella cheese, shredded
- ✓ ½ cup Parmesan cheese, grated

Directions:

1. Preheat a waffle iron and then grease it.

2. In a medium bowl, place all ingredients and mix until well combined.

3. Place ¼ of the mixture into the preheated waffle iron and cook for about 3-4 minutes or until golden brown.

4. Repeat with the remaining mixture.

5. Serve warm.

124. BROCCOLI CHAFFLES

💜 **Servings:** 2

Preparation Time: 10 Minutes

⏰ **Cooking Time:** 8 Minutes

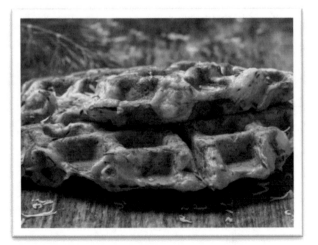

Ingredients:

- ✓ 1/3 cup raw broccoli, chopped finely
- ✓ ¼ cup Cheddar cheese, shredded
- ✓ 1 Organic egg
- ✓ ½ teaspoons garlic powder
- ✓ ½ teaspoons dried onion, minced
- ✓ Salt and freshly ground black pepper, to taste

Directions:

1. Preheat a mini waffle maker and then grease it.

2. In a medium bowl, place all ingredients and mix until well combined.

3. Place ¼ of the mixture into the preheated waffle iron and cook for about 3-4 minutes or until golden brown.

4. Repeat with the remaining mixture.

5. Serve warm.

125. CHICKEN & JALAPEÑO CHAFFLES

♥ **Servings:** 2

Preparation Time: 10 Minutes

⏰ **Cooking Time**: 10 Minutes

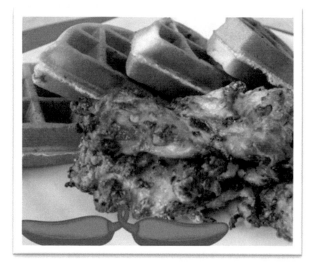

Ingredients:

- ✓ ½ cup grass-fed cooked chicken, chopped
- ✓ 1 organic egg, beaten
- ✓ ¼ cup Cheddar cheese, shredded
- ✓ 2 tablespoons Parmesan cheese, shredded
- ✓ 1 teaspoon cream cheese, softened
- ✓ 1 small jalapeño pepper, chopped
- ✓ 1/8 teaspoon onion powder
- ✓ 1/8 teaspoon garlic powder

Directions:

1. Preheat a mini waffle maker and then grease it.

2. In a medium bowl, place all the ingredients and mix until well combined.

3. Place half of the mixture into the preheated waffle iron and cook for about 4-5 minutes or until golden brown.

4. Repeat with the remaining mixture.

5. Serve warm.

Nutrition: **Calories**: 170; **Net Carbs**: 0.9g; **Fat**: 9.9g; **Saturated Fat**: 5.2g; **Carbohydrates**: 0.1g; **Dietary Fiber**: 2.6g; **Sugar**: 0.5g; **Protein**: 8.6g

126. BBQ CHICKEN CHAFFLES

♥ **Servings:** 2

Preparation Time: 10 Minutes

🕐 **Cooking Time**: 8 Minutes

Ingredients:

- ✓ 1 1/3 cups grass-fed cooked chicken, chopped
- ✓ ½ cup Cheddar cheese, shredded
- ✓ 1 tablespoon sugar-free BBQ sauce
- ✓ 1 Organic egg, beaten
- ✓ 1 tablespoon almond flour

Directions:

1. Preheat a mini waffle maker and then grease it.

2. In a bowl, place all ingredients and mix until well combined.

3. Place half of the mixture into the preheated waffle iron and cook for about four minutes or until golden brown.

4. Repeat with the remaining mixture.

5. Serve warm.

Nutrition: **Calories:** 320; **Net Carbs:** 3.6g**Fat:** 16.3g; **Saturated Fat:** 7.6g; **Carbohydrates:** 4g**Dietary Fiber:** 0.4g; **Sugar:** 2g; **Protein:** 36.9g

127. STRAWBERRY CREAM SANDWICH CHAFFLES

♥ **Servings**: 2

▨ **Preparation Time**: 10 Minutes

⏰ **Cooking Time**: 6 Minutes

Ingredients: For the Chaffles:

- ✓ 1 Large organic egg, beaten
- ✓ ½ cup mozzarella cheese, shredded finely

Filling:

- ✓ 4 teaspoons heavy cream
- ✓ 2 tablespoons powdered erythritol
- ✓ 1 teaspoon fresh lemon juice
- ✓ A pinch of fresh lemon zest, grated
- ✓ 2 fresh strawberries, hulled and sliced

Directions:

1. Preheat a mini waffle maker and then grease it.

2. For the chaffles, in a small bowl, add the egg and mozzarella cheese and stir to combine.

3. Place half of the mixture into the preheated waffle iron and cook for about 2–3 minutes.

4. Repeat with the remaining mixture.

5. Meanwhile, for the filling, in a bowl, Place all the ingredients except the strawberry slices, and with a hand mixer, beat until well combined.

6. Serve each chaffle with the cream mixture and strawberry slices.

Nutrition: **Calories**: 95; **Net Carbs**: 1.4g; **Total Fat**: 7.5g; **Saturated Fat**: 3.9g; **Cholesterol**: 110mg; **Sodium**: 82mg; **Total Carbs**: 1.7g; **Fiber**: 0.3g; **Sugar** 0.9g; **Protein**:5.5g

128. STRAWBERRY CREAM CHEESE SANDWICH CHAFFLES

💔 **Servings:** 2

Preparation Time: 15 Minutes

⏰ **Cooking Time:** 10 Minutes

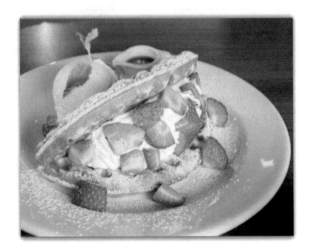

Ingredients: For the Chaffles:

- ✓ 1 Organic egg, beaten
- ✓ 1 teaspoon organic vanilla extract
- ✓ 1 tablespoon almond flour
- ✓ 1 teaspoon organic baking powder
- ✓ A pinch of ground cinnamon
- ✓ 1 cup mozzarella cheese, shredded

For the Filling:

- ✓ 2 tablespoons cream cheese, softened
- ✓ 2 tablespoons erythritol
- ✓ ¼ teaspoon organic vanilla extract
- ✓ 2 fresh strawberries, hulled and chopped

Directions:

1. Preheat a mini waffle maker and then grease it.

2. For the chaffles, in a bowl, add the egg and vanilla extract and mix well.

3. Add the flour, baking powder, and cinnamon, and mix until well combined.

4. Add the mozzarella cheese and stir to combine.

5. Place half of the mixture into the preheated waffle iron and cook for about 4–5 minutes.

6. Repeat with the remaining mixture.

7. Meanwhile, for the filling, in a bowl, Place all the ingredients except the strawberry pieces, and with a hand mixer, beat until well combined.

8. Serve each chaffle with the cream cheese mixture and strawberry pieces.

Nutrition: **Calories:** 143; **Net Carbs:**1.4 g **Total Fat:** 10.1g; **Saturated Fat:**4.5g; **Cholesterol:** 100mg; **Sodium:** 148mg; **Total Carbs:** 4.1g; **Fiber:** 0.8g; **Sugar:** 1.2g; **Protein:** 7.6g

129. BLUEBERRY PEANUT BUTTER SANDWICH CHAFFLES

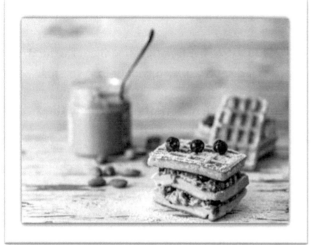

♥ **Servings:** 2

Preparation Time: 10 Minutes

⏱ **Cooking Time**: 10 Minutes

Ingredients: For the Chaffles:

- ✓ 1 Organic egg, beaten
- ✓ ½ cup cheddar cheese, shredded

For the Filling:

- ✓ 2 tablespoons erythritol
- ✓ 1 tablespoon butter, softened
- ✓ 1 tablespoon natural peanut butter
- ✓ 2 tablespoons cream cheese, softened
- ✓ ¼ teaspoon organic vanilla extract
- ✓ 2 teaspoons fresh blueberries

Directions:

1. Preheat a mini waffle maker and then grease it.

2. For the chaffles, in a small bowl, add the egg and Cheddar cheese and stir to combine.

3. Place half of the mixture into the preheated waffle iron and cook for about 3–5 minutes.

4. Repeat with the remaining mixture.

5. Meanwhile, for filling: In a medium bowl, put all ingredients and mix until well combined.

6. Serve each chaffle with the peanut butter mixture.

Nutrition: Calories: 143; **Net Carbs**: 3.3g

Total Fat: 10.1g; **Saturated Fat**: 4.5g; **Cholesterol**:100mg; **Sodium**: 148mg; **Total Carbs**: 4.1g; **Fiber**: 0.8g; **Sugar**: 1.2g; **Protein**: 7.6g

130. BERRY SAUCE
SANDWICH CHAFFLES

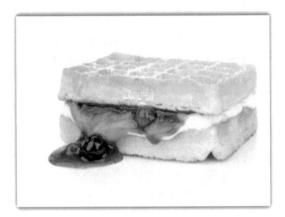

❤ **Servings:** 2

🧇 **Preparation Time**: 10 Minutes

⏰ **Cooking Time**: 8 Minutes

Ingredients: For the Filling:

- ✓ 3 Ounces frozen mixed berries, thawed with the juice
- ✓ 1 tablespoon erythritol
- ✓ 1 tablespoon water
- ✓ ¼ tablespoon fresh lemon juice
- ✓ 2 teaspoons cream

For the Chaffles:

- ✓ 1 Large organic egg, beaten
- ✓ ½ cup cheddar cheese, shredded
- ✓ 2 tablespoons almond flour

Directions:

1. For the berry sauce, add the berries in a pan, erythritol, water, and lemon juice over medium heat, and cook for about 8–10 minutes, pressing with the spoon occasionally.

2. Remove the pan of sauce from the heat and set it aside to cool before serving.

3. Preheat a mini waffle maker and then grease it.

4. In a bowl, add the egg, cheddar cheese, and almond flour and beat until well combined.

5. Place half of the mixture into the preheated waffle iron and cook for about 3–5 minutes.

6. Repeat with the remaining mixture.

7. Serve each chaffle with cream and berry sauce.

Nutrition: **Calories**: 222; **Net Carbs**: 4.7g

Total Fat: 16g; **Saturated Fat**: 7.2g; **Cholesterol**: 123mg; **Sodium**: 212mg; **Total Carbs**: 7g; **Fiber**: 2.3g; **Sugar**: 3.8g; **Protein**: 10.5g

131. CHOCOLATE SANDWICH CHAFFLES

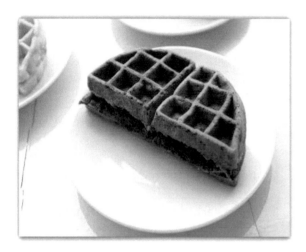

❤ **Servings**: 2

🧈 **Preparation Time**: 10 Minutes

⏱ **Cooking Time**: 10 Minutes

Ingredients: For the Chaffles:

- ✓ 1 Organic egg, beaten
- ✓ 1 Ounce cream cheese, softened
- ✓ 2 tablespoons almond flour
- ✓ 1 tablespoon cacao powder
- ✓ 2 teaspoons erythritol
- ✓ 1 teaspoon organic vanilla extract

For the Filling:

- ✓ 2 tablespoons cream cheese, softened
- ✓ 2 tablespoons erythritol
- ✓ ½ tablespoon cacao powder
- ✓ ¼ teaspoon organic vanilla extract

Directions:

1. Preheat a mini waffle maker and then grease it.

2. For the chaffles, in a medium bowl, put all ingredients and with a fork, mix until well combined.

3. Place half of the mixture into the preheated waffle iron and cook for about 3–5 minutes.

4. Repeat with the remaining mixture.

5. Meanwhile, for the filling, in a medium bowl, put all ingredients and with a hand mixer, beat until well combined.

6. Serve each chaffle with the chocolate mixture.

Nutrition: **Calories**: 192; **Net Carbs**: g

Total Fat: 16.6g; **Saturated Fat**: 7.6g; **Cholesterol**: 113mg; **Sodium**: 115mg; **Total Carbs**: 4.4g; **Fiber**: 1.9g; **Sugar**: 0.8g; **Total Protein**: 5.7g

132. EGG & BACON SANDWICH CHAFFLES

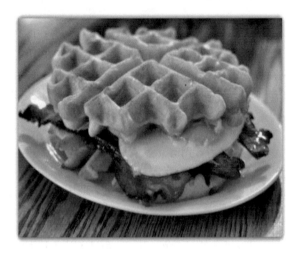

Directions:

1. Preheat a mini waffle maker and then grease it.

2. In a medium bowl, put all ingredients and with a fork, mix until well combined.

3. Place half of the mixture into the preheated waffle iron and cook for about 3–5 minutes.

4. Repeat with the remaining mixture.

5. Serve each chaffle with the filling ingredients.

❤ **Servings:** 2

Preparation Time: 10 Minutes

⏰ **Cooking Time:** 20 Minutes

Nutrition: Calories: 197; Total Fat: 14.5g

Saturated Fat:4.1g; Cholesterol: 267mg; Sodium: 224g; Total Carbs: 2.7g; Fiber: 0.8g; Sugar: 0.8g; Protein: 12.9g

Ingredients: For the Chaffles:

- ✓ 2 large organic eggs, beaten
- ✓ 4 tablespoons almond flour
- ✓ 1 teaspoon organic baking powder
- ✓ 1 cup mozzarella cheese, shredded

For the Filling:

- ✓ 4 Organic fried eggs
- ✓ 4 Cooked bacon slices

133. TOMATO SANDWICH CHAFFLES

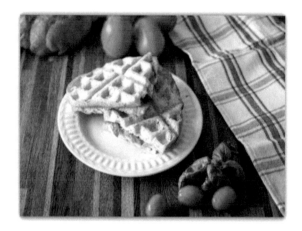

💟 **Servings:** 2

🧇 **Preparation Time:** 5 Minutes

⏰ **Cooking Time:** 6 Minutes

Ingredients: For the Chaffles:

- ✓ 1 large organic egg, beaten
- ✓ ½ cup Colby jack cheese, shredded finely
- ✓ 1/8 teaspoon organic vanilla extract

For the Filling:

- ✓ 1 small tomato, sliced
- ✓ 2 teaspoons fresh basil leaves

Directions:

1. Preheat a mini waffle maker and then grease it.

2. For the chaffles, in a small bowl, place all the ingredients and stir to combine.

3. Place half of the mixture into the preheated waffle iron and cook for about 3 minutes.

4. Repeat with the remaining mixture.

5. Serve each chaffle with tomato slices and basil leaves.

> **Nutrition: Calories:** 155; **Net Carbs:** 2.4g
>
> **Total Fat:** 11.6g; **Saturated Fat:** 6.8g; **Cholesterol:** 118mg; **Sodium:** 217mg; **Total Carbs:** 3g; **Fiber:** 0.6g; **Sugar:** 1.4g; **Protein:** 9.6g

134. CHICKEN SANDWICH CHAFFLES

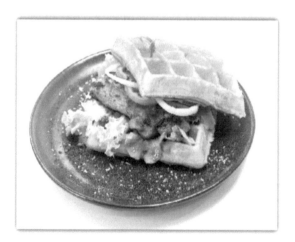

💟 **Servings:** 2

🧇 **Preparation Time:** 10 Minutes

⏰ **Cooking Time:** 8 Minutes

Ingredients: For the Chaffles:

- ✓ 1 Large organic egg, beaten
- ✓ ½ cup cheddar cheese, shredded
- ✓ A pinch of salt and ground black pepper

For the Filling:

- ✓ 1 (6-ounce) cooked chicken breast, halved
- ✓ 2 Lettuce leaves
- ✓ ¼ of a small onion, sliced
- ✓ 1 small tomato, sliced

Directions:

1. Preheat a mini waffle maker and then grease it.

2. For the chaffles, in a medium bowl, put all ingredients and with a fork, mix until well combined.

3. Place half of the mixture into the preheated waffle iron and cook for about 3–4 minutes.

4. Repeat with the remaining mixture.

5. Serve each chaffle with the filling ingredients.

Nutrition: **Calories:** 259; **Net Carbs:** 2.5g **Total Fat:** 14.1g; **Saturated Fat:** 6.8g **Cholesterol:** 177mg; **Sodium:** 334mg; **Total Carbs:** 3.3g; **Fiber:** 0.8g; **Sugar:** 2g; **Protein:** 28.7g

135. PORK SANDWICH CHAFFLES

♥ **Servings:** 2

Preparation Time: 15 Minutes

⏰ **Cooking Time:** 16 Minutes

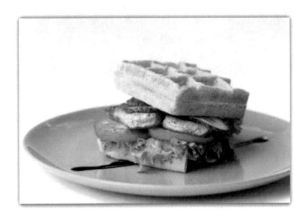

Ingredients: For the Chaffles:

- ✓ 2 Large organic eggs
- ✓ ¼ cup superfine blanched almond flour
- ✓ ¾ teaspoon organic baking powder
- ✓ ½ teaspoon garlic powder
- ✓ 1 cup cheddar cheese, shredded

For the Filling:

- ✓ 12 Ounces cooked pork, cut into slices
- ✓ 1 Tomato, sliced
- ✓ 4 Lettuce leaves

Directions:

1. Preheat a mini waffle maker and then grease it.

2. For the chaffles, in a bowl, add the eggs,

almond flour, baking powder, and garlic powder, and beat until well combined.

3. Add the cheese and stir to combine.

4. Place ¼ of the mixture into the preheated waffle iron and cook for about 3–4 minutes.

5. Repeat with the remaining mixture.

6. Serve each chaffle with the filling ingredients.

Nutrition: **Calories**: 319; **Net Carbs**: 2.5g

Total Fat: 18.2g; **Saturated Fat**: 8g; **Cholesterol**: 185mg; **Sodium**: 263mg; **Total Carbs**: 3.5g; **Fiber**: 1g; **Sugar**: 0.9g; **Protein**: 34.2g

136. HAM SANDWICH CHAFFLES

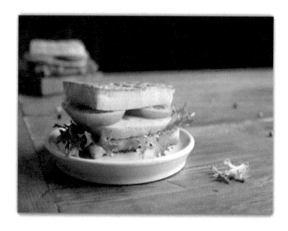

❤ **Servings**: 2

🧇 **Preparation Time**: 10 Minutes

⏰ **Cooking Time**: 8 Minutes

Ingredients:

✓ 1 organic egg, beaten
✓ ½ cup Monterrey Jack cheese, shredded
✓ 1 teaspoon coconut flour
✓ A pinch of garlic powder

For the Filling:

✓ 2 sugar-free ham slices
✓ 1 small tomato, sliced
✓ 2 lettuce leaves

Directions:

1. Preheat a mini waffle maker and then grease it.

2. For the chaffles, in a medium bowl, put all ingredients and with a fork, mix until well combined.

3. Place half of the mixture into the preheated waffle iron and cook for about 3–4 minutes.

4. Repeat with the remaining mixture.

5. Serve each chaffle with the filling ingredients.

Nutrition: **Calories**: 156; **Net Carbs**: 3.7g

Total Fat: 8.7g; **Saturated Fat**: 3.4g; **Cholesterol** 114mg; **Sodium**: 794mg; **Total Carbs**: 5.5g; **Fiber**: 1.8g; **Sugar**: 1.5g; **Protein**: 13.9g

137. SALMON & CHEESE SANDWICH CHAFFLES

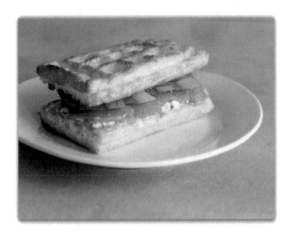

💜 **Servings**: 2

🧇 **Preparation Time**: 15 Minutes

⏰ **Cooking Time**: 24 Minutes

Ingredients: For the Chaffles:

- ✓ 2 Organic eggs
- ✓ ½ Ounce butter, melted
- ✓ 1 cup mozzarella cheese, shredded
- ✓ 2 tablespoons almond flour
- ✓ A pinch of salt

For the Filling:

- ✓ ½ cup smoked salmon
- ✓ 1/3 cup avocado, peeled, pitted, and sliced
- ✓ 2 tablespoons feta cheese, crumbled

Directions:

1. Preheat a mini waffle maker and then grease it.

2. For the chaffles, in a medium bowl, put all ingredients and with a fork, mix until well combined.

3. Place ¼ of the mixture into the preheated waffle iron and cook for about 5–6 minutes.

4. Repeat with the remaining mixture.

5. Serve each chaffle with the filling ingredients.

Nutrition: **Calories**: 169; **Net Carbs**: 1.2g

Total Fat: 13.5g; **Saturated Fat**: 5g

Cholesterol: 101mg; **Sodium**: 319mg

Total Carbs: 2.8g; **Fiber**: 1.6g; **Sugar**: 0.6g

Protein: 8.9g

138. SALMON & CREAM SANDWICH CHAFFLES

💜 **Servings**: 2

🧇 **Preparation Time**: 10 Minutes

⏰ **Cooking Time**: 8 Minutes

Ingredients: For the Chaffles:

- ✓ 1 Organic egg, beaten
- ✓ ½ cup cheddar cheese, shredded
- ✓ 1 tablespoon almond flour
- ✓ 1 tablespoon fresh rosemary, chopped

For the Filling:

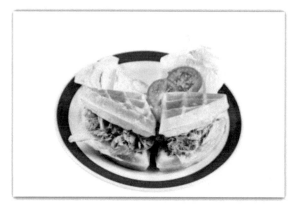

- ✓ ¼ cup smoked salmon
- ✓ 1 teaspoon fresh dill, chopped
- ✓ 2 tablespoons cream

Directions:

1. Preheat a mini waffle maker and then grease it.

2. For the chaffles, in a medium bowl, put all ingredients and with a fork, mix until well combined.

3. Place half of the mixture into the preheated waffle iron and cook for about 3–4 minutes.

4. Repeat with the remaining mixture.

5. Serve each chaffle with the filling ingredients.

Nutrition: Calories: 202; **Net Carbs**: 1.7g

Total Fat: 15.1g; **Saturated Fat**: 7.5g

Cholesterol: 118mg; **Sodium**: 345mg

Total Carbs: 2.9g; **Fiber**: 1.2g; **Sugar**: 0.7g

Protein: 13.2g

139. TUNA SANDWICH CHAFFLES

❤ **Servings:** 2

🧇 **Preparation Time**: 10 Minutes

⏰ **Cooking Time**: 8 Minutes

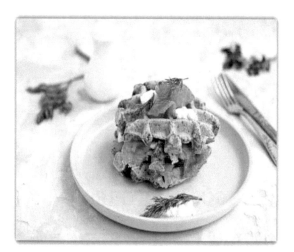

Ingredients: For the Chaffles:

- ✓ 1 Organic egg, beaten
- ✓ ½ cup cheddar cheese, shredded
- ✓ 1 tablespoon almond flour
- ✓ A pinch of salt

For the Filling:

- ✓ ¼ cup water-packed tuna, flaked
- ✓ 2 Lettuce leaves

Directions:

1. Preheat a mini waffle maker and then grease it.

2. For the chaffles, in a medium bowl, put all ingredients and with a fork, mix until well combined.

3. Place half of the mixture into the preheated waffle iron and cook for about 3–4 minutes.

4. Repeat with the remaining mixture.

5. Serve each chaffle with the filling ingredients.

> **Nutrition:** **Calories:** 186; **Total Fat:** 13.6g
>
> **Saturated Fat:** 6.8g; **Cholesterol:** 120mg; **Sodium:** 342mg; **Total Carbs:** 1.3g; **Fiber:** 0.4g; **Sugar:** 0.5g; **Protein:** 13.6g

140. CHOCOLATE OREO SANDWICH CHAFFLES

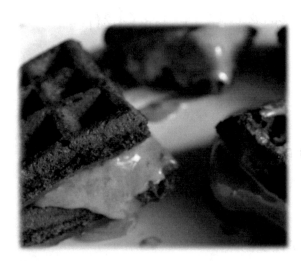

 Servings: 2

 Preparation Time: 0 Minutes

 Cooking Time: 5 Minutes

Ingredients: For the Chaffles:

- ✓ 1 Organic egg
- ✓ 1 tablespoon heavy cream
- ✓ 2 tablespoons Erythritol
- ✓ 1½ tablespoons cacao powder
- ✓ 1 teaspoon coconut flour
- ✓ 2 tablespoons Erythritol
- ✓ ½ teaspoon organic baking powder
- ✓ ½ teaspoon organic vanilla extract

For the Filling:

- ✓ 3 tablespoons mascarpone cheese, softened
- ✓ 2 tablespoons heavy whipping cream
- ✓ ½ teaspoon organic vanilla extract
- ✓ 2 tablespoons powdered Erythritol

Directions:

1. Preheat a mini waffle maker and then grease it.

2. For the chaffles, in a medium bowl, put all ingredients and with a fork, mix until well combined.

3. Place half of the mixture into the preheated waffle iron and cook for about 3-5 minutes.

4. Repeat with the remaining mixture.

5. Meanwhile, for the filling, in a bowl, add all ingredients and mix well.

6. Spread the filling mixture over one chaffle and top with the remaining chaffle.

7. Cut in half and serve.

> **Nutrition:** **Calories:** 168; **Net Carbs:** 3.2g; **Fat:** 14.4g; **Carbohydrates:** 5g; **Dietary Fiber:** 1.7g; **Sugar:** 0.4g; **Protein:** 6.8g

141. PEANUT BUTTER SANDWICH CHAFFLES

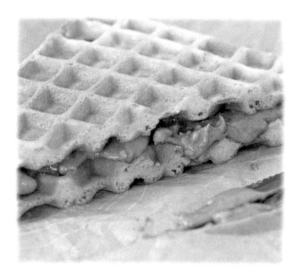

❤ **Servings**: 2

🧇 **Preparation Time**: 10 Minutes

⏰ **Cooking Time**: 10 Minutes

Ingredients: For the Chaffles:

- ✓ 1 Organic egg, beaten
- ✓ 2 tablespoons almond flour
- ✓ ½ teaspoon organic baking powder
- ✓ ½ cup Mozzarella cheese, shredded

For the Filling:

- ✓ 2 tablespoons natural peanut butter
- ✓ 2 tablespoons heavy cream
- ✓ 2 teaspoons powdered Erythritol

Directions:

1. Preheat a mini waffle maker and then grease it.

2. For the chaffles, in a medium bowl, add all ingredients, and with a fork, mix until well combined.

3. Place half of the mixture into the preheated waffle iron and cook for about 3-5 minutes.

4. Repeat with the remaining mixture.

5. Meanwhile, for the filling, in a bowl, add all ingredients and mix well.

6. Spread the peanut butter mixture over one chaffle and top with the remaining chaffle.

7. Cut in half and serve.

Nutrition: **Calories**: 243; **Net Carbs**: 4.1g; **Fat**: 20.8g; **Carbohydrates**: 5.8g; **Dietary Fiber**: 1.7g; **Sugar**: 1.9g; **Protein**: 9.1g

142. PEANUT BUTTER & JAM SANDWICH CHAFFLES

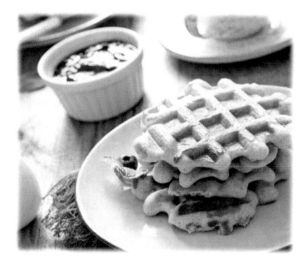

Servings: 2

Preparation Time: 10 Minutes

Cooking Time: 8 Minutes

Ingredients: For the Chaffles:

- ✓ 1 Organic egg
- ✓ ½ cup Monterey Jack cheese, shredded
- ✓ 1 tablespoon almond flour

For the Filling:

- ✓ 1 tablespoon peanut butter
- ✓ 1 tablespoon sugar-free Strawberry jam

Directions:

1. Preheat a mini waffle maker and then grease it.

2. For the chaffles, in a medium bowl, add all ingredients, and with a fork, mix until well combined.

3. Place half of the mixture into the preheated waffle iron and cook for about 3-4 minutes.

4. Spread the peanut butter and jam over one chaffle and top with the remaining chaffle.

5. Cut in half and serve.

Nutrition: **Calories:** 206; **Net Carbs:** 6.6g**Fat:** 16.7g; **Carbohydrates:** 2.6g; **Dietary Fiber:** 0.9g; **Sugar:** 1.2g; **Protein:** 11.7g

143. BLUEBERRY SANDWICH CHAFFLES

Servings: 2

Preparation Time: 10 Minutes

Cooking Time: 10 Minutes

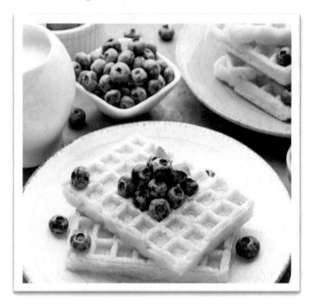

Ingredients:

- ✓ 1 Organic egg, beaten
- ✓ ½ cup Cheddar cheese, shredded

For the Filling:

- ✓ 2 tablespoons Erythritol
- ✓ 1 tablespoon butter, softened
- ✓ 1 tablespoon natural peanut butter
- ✓ 2 tablespoons cream cheese, softened
- ✓ ¼ teaspoon organic vanilla extract
- ✓ 2 teaspoons fresh blueberries

Directions:

1. Preheat a mini waffle maker and then grease it.

2. For the chaffles, in a small bowl, add the egg and Cheddar cheese and stir to combine.

3. Place half of the mixture into the preheated waffle iron and cook for about 3-5 minutes.

4. Repeat with the remaining mixture.

5. Meanwhile, for the filling, in a medium bowl, add all ingredients and mix until well combined.

6. Place the filling mixture over one chaffle and top with the remaining chaffle.

7. Cut in half and serve.

Nutrition: **Calories**: 143; **Net Carbs**: 3.3g; **Fat**: 10.1g; **Carbohydrates**: 4.1g; **Dietary Fiber**: 0.8g; **Sugar**: 1.2g; **Protein**: 7.6g

144. BLACKBERRY RICOTTA CHAFFLES

❤ **Servings**: 2

▨ **Preparation Time**: 5 Minutes

⏰ **Cooking Time**: 5 Minutes

Ingredients: For the Chaffles:

✓ 2 Large organic eggs
✓ 1 cup Mozzarella cheese, shredded finely

For the Filling:

✓ ¼ cup fresh blackberries
✓ 4 teaspoons ricotta cheese, crumbled

Directions:

1. Preheat a mini waffle maker and then grease it.

2. For the chaffles, in a bowl, add the eggs and cheese and stir to combine.

3. Place ¼ of the mixture into the preheated waffle iron and cook for about 3-4 minutes.

4. Repeat with the remaining mixture.

5. Place the filling ingredients over two chaffles and top with remaining chaffles.

6. Cut each in half and serve.

Nutrition: **Calories**: 67; **Net Carbs**: 1.1g; **Fat**: 4.2g; **Carbohydrates**: 1.6g; **Dietary Fiber**: 0.5g; **Sugar**: 0.7g; **Protein**: 5.9g

145. RASPBERRY SANDWICH CHAFFLES

Servings: 2

Preparation Time: 15 Minutes

Cooking Time: 10 Minutes

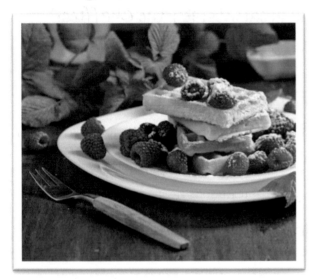

Ingredients: For the Chaffles:

- ✓ 1 Organic egg, beaten
- ✓ 1 teaspoon organic vanilla extract
- ✓ 1 tablespoon almond flour
- ✓ 1 teaspoon organic baking powder
- ✓ A pinch of ground cinnamon
- ✓ 1 cup Mozzarella cheese, shredded

For the Filling:

- ✓ 2 tablespoons cream cheese, softened
- ✓ 2 tablespoons Erythritol
- ✓ ¼ teaspoon organic vanilla extract
- ✓ 4 Fresh raspberries, chopped

Directions:

1. Preheat a mini waffle maker and then grease it.

2. For the chaffles, in a bowl, add the egg and vanilla extract and mix well.

3. Add the flour, baking powder, and cinnamon and mix until well combined.

4. Add the Mozzarella cheese and stir to combine.

5. Place half of the mixture into the preheated waffle iron and cook for about 4-5 minutes.

6. Repeat with the remaining mixture.

7. Meanwhile, for the filling, in a bowl, place all the ingredients except the strawberry pieces, and with a hand mixer, beat until well combined.

8. Spread cream cheese mixture over one chaffle and top with raspberries.

9. Cover with remaining chaffle.

10. Cut in half and serve.

Nutrition: **Calories**: 143; **Net Carbs**: 6.6g; **Fat**: 10.1g; **Carbohydrates**: 4.1g; **Dietary Fiber**: 0.8g; **Sugar**: 1.2g; **Protein**: 0.8g

146. BERRIES SAUCE SANDWICH CHAFFLES

💗 **Servings:** 2

🧇 **Preparation Time:** 10 Minutes

⏰ **Cooking Time:** 8 Minutes

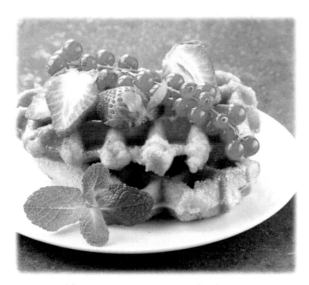

Ingredients: For the Filling:

- ✓ 3 Ounces frozen mixed berries, thawed with the juice
- ✓ 1 tablespoon Erythritol
- ✓ 1 tablespoon water
- ✓ ¼ tablespoon fresh lemon juice
- ✓ 2 teaspoons cream

For the Chaffles:

- ✓ 1 Large organic egg, beaten
- ✓ ½ cup Cheddar cheese, shredded
- ✓ 2 tablespoons almond flour

Directions:

1. For the berry sauce, in a pan, add the berries, Erythritol, water, and lemon juice over medium heat and cook for about 8-10 minutes, pressing with the spoon occasionally.

2. Remove the pan of sauce from the heat and set it aside to cool before serving.

3. Preheat a mini waffle maker and then grease it.

4. In a bowl, add the egg, Cheddar cheese, and almond flour and beat until well combined.

5. Place half of the mixture into the preheated waffle iron and cook for about 3-5 minutes.

6. Repeat with the remaining mixture.

7. Spread berry sauce over one chaffle and top with the remaining chaffle.

8. Cut in half and serve.

Nutrition: **Calories:** 222; **Net Carbs:** 4.7g; **Fat:** 21.5g; **Carbohydrates:** 7g; **Dietary Fiber:** 2.3g; **Sugar:** 3.8g; **Protein:** 10.5g

147. GRILLED CHEESE SANDWICH CHAFFLES

♥ **Servings:** 2

Preparation Time: 0 Minutes

⏰ **Cooking Time**: 5 Minutes

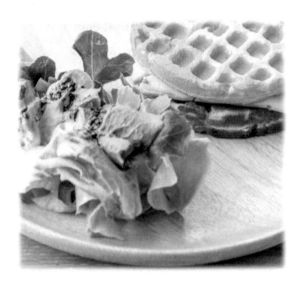

Ingredients: For the Chaffles:

- ✓ 1 Organic egg
- ✓ ½ cup Cheddar cheese, shredded
- ✓ ¼ teaspoon garlic powder

For the Filling:

- ✓ 1 tablespoon butter
- ✓ ¼ cup Cheddar cheese, shredded

Directions:

1. Preheat a mini waffle maker and then grease it.

2. In a bowl, add the egg, Cheddar cheese, and almond flour and beat until well combined.

3. Place half of the mixture into the preheated waffle iron and cook for about 3-4 minutes.

4. Repeat with the remaining mixture.

5. In a frying pan, melt the butter over medium heat.

6. Cover with the second chaffle and cook for about 1 minute per side.

7. Transfer the chaffle sandwich onto a plate and cut it in half.

8. Serve immediately.

Nutrition: **Calories**: 254; **Net Carbs**: 1g; **Fat**: 22g; **Carbohydrates**: 1g; **Dietary Fiber**: 0g; **Sugar**: 0.5g; **Protein**: 13.4g

148. BACON & EGG SANDWICH CHAFFLES

♥ **Servings:** 2

Preparation Time: 10 Minutes

⏰ **Cooking Time**: 20 Minutes

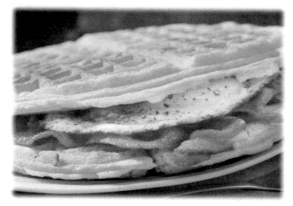

Ingredients: For the Chaffles:

- ✓ 2 large organic eggs, beaten
- ✓ 4 tablespoons almond flour
- ✓ 1 teaspoon organic baking powder
- ✓ 1 cup Mozzarella cheese, shredded

For the Filling:

- ✓ 4 Organic fried eggs
- ✓ 4 Cooked bacon slices

Directions:

1. Preheat a mini waffle maker and then grease it.

2. For the chaffles, in a medium bowl, add all ingredients, and with a fork, mix until well combined.

3. Place half of the mixture into the preheated waffle iron and cook for about 3-5 minutes.

4. Repeat with the remaining mixture.

5. Place the filling ingredients over one chaffle and top with the remaining chaffle.

6. Cut each in half and serve.

Nutrition: **Calories:** 197; **Net Carbs:** 1.9g **Fat:** 14.5g; **Carbohydrates:** 2.7g; **Dietary Fiber:**0.8g; **Sugar:** 0.7g; **Protein:** 15.7g

149. BACON & LETTUCE SANDWICH CHAFFLES

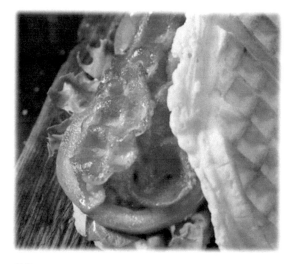

♥ **Servings:** 2

Preparation Time: 10 Minutes

⏰ **Cooking Time**: 8 Minutes

Ingredients: For the Chaffles:

- ✓ 1 Organic egg
- ✓ ½ cup Mozzarella cheese, shredded
- ✓ 1 tablespoon scallion, chopped
- ✓ ½ teaspoon Italian seasoning

For the Filling:

- ✓ 2 Lettuce leaves
- ✓ 2 Cooked bacon slices
- ✓ 2 Tomato slices

Directions:

1. Preheat a mini waffle maker and then grease it.

2. For the chaffles, in a medium bowl, add all ingredients, and with a fork, mix until well combined.

3. Place half of the mixture into the preheated waffle iron and cook for about 4 minutes.

4. Repeat with the remaining mixture.

5. Place the lettuce, bacon, and tomato slices over one chaffle and top with the remaining chaffle.

6. Cut in half and serve.

Nutrition: Calories: 216; **Net Carbs:** 1.5g; **Fat:** 16g; **Carbohydrates:** 1.8g; **Dietary Fiber:** 0.3g; **Sugar:** 0.7g; **Protein:** 15.7g

150. BACON & CHEESE CHAFFLES

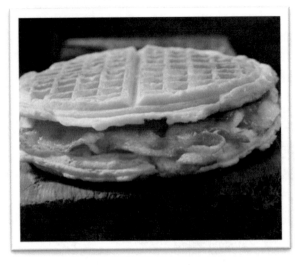

💗 **Servings:** 2

Preparation Time: 10 Minutes

⏰ **Cooking Time:** 8 Minutes

Ingredients: For the Chaffles:

- ✓ 1 Organic egg
- ✓ ½ cup Mozzarella cheese, shredded
- ✓ 2 tablespoons almond flour

For the Filling:

- ✓ 2 Cooked bacon slices
- ✓ 1 Cheddar cheese slice

Directions:

1. Preheat a mini waffle maker and then grease it.

2. For the chaffles, in a medium bowl, add all ingredients, and with a fork, mix until well combined.

3. Place half of the mixture into the

preheated waffle iron and cook for about 3-4 minutes.

4. Repeat with the remaining mixture.

5. Place the bacon and cheese slices over the chaffle and top with the remaining chaffle.

6. Cut in half and serve.

> **Nutrition:** **Calories:** 310; **Net Carbs:** 1.5g; **Fat:** 24g; **Carbohydrates:** 2.3g; **Dietary Fiber:** 0.8g; **Sugar:** 0.5g; **Protein:** 19g

151. HAM & CHEESE CHAFFLES

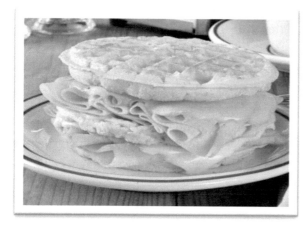

♥ **Servings:** 2

Preparation Time: 10 Minutes

⏱ **Cooking Time:** 8 Minutes

Ingredients: For the Chaffles:

- ✓ 1 large organic egg
- ✓ ½ cup cheddar cheese, shredded
- ✓ 3 tablespoons almond flour
- ✓ ¼ teaspoon organic baking powder

For the Filling:

- ✓ 1-2 tablespoons mayonnaise
- ✓ 1 Sugar-free ham slice
- ✓ 1 Cheddar cheese slice

Directions:

1. Preheat a mini waffle maker and then grease it.

2. For the chaffles, in a medium bowl, add all ingredients, and with a fork, mix until well combined.

3. Place half of the mixture into the preheated waffle iron and cook for about 3-4 minutes.

4. Repeat with the remaining mixture.

5. Spread mayonnaise over one chaffle.

6. Place the ham and cheese slice over the chaffle and top with the remaining chaffle.

7. Cut in half and serve.

> **Nutrition:** **Calories:** 273; **Net Carbs:** 2.7g; **Fat:** 21.2g; **Carbohydrates:** 4.1g; **Dietary Fiber:** 1.4g; **Sugar:** 0.7g; **Protein:** 14g

6. Cut in half and serve.

152. HAM & TOMATO SANDWICH CHAFFLES

♥ **Servings**: 2

Preparation Time: 10 Minutes

⏰ **Cooking Time**: 8 Minutes

Ingredients: For the Chaffles:

- ✓ 1 organic egg, beaten
- ✓ ½ cup Monterrey Jack cheese, shredded
- ✓ 1 teaspoon coconut flour
- ✓ A pinch of garlic powder

For the Filling:

- ✓ 2 sugar-free ham slices
- ✓ 1 small tomato, sliced
- ✓ 2 lettuce leaves

Directions:

1. Preheat a mini waffle maker and then grease it.

2. For the chaffles, in a medium bowl, add all ingredients, and with a fork, mix until well combined.

3. Place half of the mixture into the preheated waffle iron and cook for about 3-4 minutes.

4. Repeat with the remaining mixture.

5. Place the filling ingredients over one chaffle and top with the remaining chaffle.

153. SMOKED SALMON & CREAM SANDWICH CHAFFLES

♥ **Servings**: 2

Preparation Time: 10 Minutes

⏰ **Cooking Time**: 8 Minutes

Ingredients: For the Chaffles:

- ✓ 1 Organic egg, beaten
- ✓ ½ cup Cheddar cheese, shredded
- ✓ 1 tablespoon almond flour
- ✓ 1 tablespoon fresh rosemary, chopped

For the Filling:

- ✓ ¼ cup smoked salmon
- ✓ 1 teaspoon fresh dill, chopped
- ✓ 2 tablespoons cream

Directions:

1. Preheat a mini waffle maker and then grease it.

2. For the chaffles, in a medium bowl, add all ingredients, and with a fork, mix until well combined.

3. Place half of the mixture into the preheated waffle iron and cook for about 3-4 minutes.

4. Repeat with the remaining mixture.

5. Place the filling ingredients over one chaffle and top with the remaining chaffle.

6. Cut in half and serve.

Nutrition: **Calories**: 202; **Net Carbs**: 1.7g

Fat: 15.1g; **Carbohydrates**: 2.9g; **Dietary Fiber**: 1.2g; **Sugar**: 0.7g; **Protein**: 13.2g

154. SMOKED SALMON & FETA SANDWICH CHAFFLES

💗 **Servings**: 2

🍰 **Preparation Time**: 15 Minutes

⏰ **Cooking Time**: 24 Minutes

Ingredients: For the Chaffles:

- ✓ 2 Organic eggs
- ✓ ½ Ounce butter, melted
- ✓ 1 cup Mozzarella cheese, shredded
- ✓ 2 tablespoons almond flour
- ✓ A pinch of salt

For the Filling:

- ✓ ½ cup smoked salmon
- ✓ 1/3 cup avocado, peeled, pitted, and sliced
- ✓ 2 tablespoons feta cheese, crumbled

Directions:

1. Preheat a mini waffle maker and then grease it.

2. For the chaffles, in a medium bowl, add all ingredients, and with a fork, mix until well combined.

3. Place ¼ of the mixture into the preheated waffle iron and cook for about 5-6 minutes.

4. Repeat with the remaining mixture.

5. Place the filling ingredients over two chaffles and top with the remaining chaffles.

6. Cut each in half and serve.

Nutrition: **Calories**: 169; **Net Carbs**: 1.2g; **Fat**: 13.5g; **Carbohydrates**: 2.8g; **Dietary Fiber**: 1.6g; **Sugar**: 1.6g; **Protein**: 8.9g

155. CHAFFLE TACOS

🫀 **Servings:** 2

🧇 **Preparation Time:** 10 Minutes

⏰ **Cooking Time:** 15 Minutes

Ingredients: For the Chaffle:

- ✓ 2 tablespoons coconut flour
- ✓ 3 eggs (beaten)
- ✓ ½ cup shredded mozzarella cheese
- ✓ ½ cup shredded cheddar cheese
- ✓ A pinch of salt
- ✓ ½ teaspoon oregano

For the Taco Filling:

- ✓ 1 Garlic clove (minced)
- ✓ 1 Small onion (finely chopped)
- ✓ ½ Pound ground beef
- ✓ 1 teaspoon olive oil
- ✓ 1 teaspoon cumin
- ✓ ½ teaspoon Italian seasoning
- ✓ 1 teaspoon paprika
- ✓ 1 teaspoon chili powder
- ✓ 1 Roma tomato (diced)
- ✓ 1 green bell pepper (diced)
- ✓ 4 tablespoons sour cream
- ✓ 1 tablespoon chopped green onions

Directions:

1. Plug the waffle maker to preheat it and spray it with a non-stick cooking spray.

2. In a mixing bowl, combine the mozzarella cheese, cheddar, coconut flour, salt, and oregano. Add the eggs and mix until the ingredients are well combined.

3. Fill the waffle maker with an appropriate amount of batter. Spread the mixture to the edges to cover all the holes on the waffle maker.

4. Close the waffle maker and cook for about 5 minutes or according to the waffle maker's settings.

5. After the cooking cycle, use a plastic or silicone utensil to remove the chaffle from the waffle maker. Set aside.

6. Repeat steps 3 to 5 until you have cooked all the batter into chaffles.

7. Heat a large skillet over medium to high heat.

8. Transfer the beef to a paper towel-lined plate to drain and wipe the skillet clean.

9. Add the olive oil and leave it to get hot.

10. Add the onions and garlic and sauté for 3-4 minutes or until the onion is translucent, stirring often.

11. Add the diced tomatoes and green pepper—Cook for 1 minute.

12. Add the browned ground beef. Stir in the cumin, paprika, chili powder, and Italian

seasoning.

13. Reduce the heat and cook on low for about 8 minutes, often stirring to prevent burning.

14. Remove the skillet from heat.

15. Scoop the taco mixture into the chaffles and top with chopped green onion and sour cream.

16. Enjoy.

Nutrition: **Calories**: 321 %; **Daily Value Total Fat**: 17.5g 22%; **Saturated Fat**: 8.5g 43%; **Cholesterol**: 196mg 65%; **Sodium**: 266mg 12%; **Total Carbohydrates**: 12.6g 5%; **Dietary Fiber**: 4.4g 16%; **Total Sugars**: 4.5g; **Protein**: 28.6g; **Vitamin D**: 13mcg 66%; **Calcium**: 156mg 12%; **Iron**: 13mg 74%; **Potassium**: 533mg 11%

156. CHICKEN PARMESAN CHAFFLE

Servings: 2

Preparation Time: 5 Minutes

Cooking Time: 13 Minutes

Ingredients:

- ✓ 1 egg (beaten)
- ✓ ½ cup shredded chicken
- ✓ 2 tablespoons shredded parmesan cheese
- ✓ 1/3 cup shredded mozzarella cheese
- ✓ ¼ teaspoon garlic powder
- ✓ ¼ teaspoon onion powder
- ✓ 2 tablespoons marinara sauce
- ✓ 1 teaspoon Italian seasoning

For the Garnish:

- ✓ 1 tablespoon chopped green onions

Directions:

1. Plug the waffle maker to preheat it and spray it with a non-stick cooking spray.

2. In a mixing bowl, combine the mozzarella cheese, shredded chicken, Italian seasoning, onion powder, and garlic powder. Add the egg and mix until the ingredients are well combined.

3. Pour half of the batter into the waffle maker and spread out the mixture to the edges to cover all the holes on the waffle maker.

4. Close the waffle maker and cook for about four minutes or according to your waffle maker's settings.

5. Meanwhile, preheat your oven to 400°F and line a baking sheet with parchment paper.

6. After the cooking cycle, use a plastic or silicone utensil to remove the chaffle from the waffle maker.

7. Repeat 3, 4, and 6 to make the second chaffle.

8. Spread marinara sauce over the surface

of both chaffles and sprinkle the parmesan cheese over the chaffles.

9. Arrange the chaffles into the baking sheet and place them in the oven—Bake for about 5 minutes or until the cheese melts.

10. Remove the chaffles from the oven and let them cool for a few minutes.

11. Serve and top with chopped green onion.

Nutrition: Calories:144 %; **Daily Value Total**

Fat:6.7g 9%; **Saturated Fat**: 2.7g 14%; **Cholesterol**: 118mg 39%; **Sodium**: 212mg 9%; **Total Carbohydrates**: 3.7g 1%; **Dietary Fiber**: 0.5g 2%; **Total Sugars**: 2g; **Protein**: 16.9g **Vitamin D**: 8mcg 39%; **Calcium**: 89mg 7%; **Iron** 1mg 5%; **Potassium**: 160mg 3%

---

157. BROCCOLI AND CHEESE CHAFFLE

❤ **Servings:** 1

🧇 **Preparation Time**: 5 Minutes

⏰ **Cooking Time**: 15 Minutes

Ingredients:

- ✓ 1/3 cup broccoli (finely chopped)
- ✓ ½ teaspoon oregano
- ✓ 1/8 teaspoon salt or to taste
- ✓ 1/8 teaspoon ground black pepper or to taste
- ✓ ½ teaspoon garlic powder
- ✓ ½ teaspoon onion powder
- ✓ 1 egg (beaten)
- ✓ 4 tablespoons shredded cheddar cheese

Directions:

1. Plug the waffle maker to preheat it and spray it with a non-stick cooking spray.

2. In a mixing bowl, combine the cheese, oregano, pepper, garlic, salt, and onion. Add the egg and mix until the ingredients are well combined.

3. Fold in the chopped broccoli.

4. Pour an appropriate amount of the batter into your waffle maker and spread out the mixture to the edges to cover all the holes on the waffle maker.

5. Cook time may vary in some waffle makers.

6. After the cooking cycle, use a silicone or plastic utensil to remove the chaffle from the waffle maker.

7. Repeat steps 4 to 6 until you have cooked all the batter into chaffles.

8. Serve and top with sour cream as desired.

Nutrition: **Calories**: 198%; **Daily Value Total**

Fat: 13.9g 18%; **Saturated Fat**: 7.3g 37%; **Cholesterol**: 193mg 64%; **Sodium**: 539mg 23%; **Total Carbohydrates**: 5.2g 2%; **Dietary Fiber**: 1.3g 5%; **Total Sugars**: 1.8g; **Protein**: 13.9g; **Vitamin D**: 19mcg 94%; **Calcium**: 259mg 20%; **Iron**: 2mg 10%; **Potassium**: 222mg 5%

---

158. SIMPLE CORNBREAD CHAFFLE

❤ **Servings:** 2

🍳 **Preparation Time**: 4 Minutes

⏰ **Cooking Time**: 10 Minutes

Ingredients:

- ✓ 4 eggs
- ✓ 1 cup cheddar cheese, shredded
- ✓ 8 Slices jalapeno, optional
- ✓ 1 teaspoon red hot sauce
- ✓ ¼ teaspoon low carb corn extract
- ✓ Pinch salt

Directions:

1. Preheat the waffle maker.

2. Crack the eggs in a small bowl and whip.

3. Add all the other ingredients and mix thoroughly.

4. Add a pinch of shredded cheese to the hot waffle maker—cook for 30 seconds.

5. Pour half of the egg mixture into the preheated waffle maker.

6. Cook for 5 minutes.

7. Remove, allow to cool, and enjoy.

Nutrition: **Calories**: 155 Cal; **Total Fat**: 12g; **Saturated Fat**: 0g; **Cholesterol**: 0mg; **Sodium**: 0mg; **Total Carbs**: 1.2g; **Fiber**: 0g; **Sugar**: 0g; **Protein**: 10g

159. TUNA CHAFFLES

❤ **Servings**: 2

🍳 **Preparation Time**: 5 Minutes

⏰ **Cooking Time**: 8 Minutes

Ingredients:

- ✓ 1 Packet of tuna, drained
- ✓ ½ cup mozzarella cheese
- ✓ 1 egg
- ✓ A pinch of salt

Directions:

1. Preheat the waffle maker

2. Whip the egg in a small mixing bowl.

3. Add the tuna, cheese, and season with the salt. Mix well.

4. For a crispy crust, add a teaspoon of shredded cheese to the waffle maker and cook for 30 seconds.

5. Pour half of the mixture into the mini waffle maker and cook for 4 minutes.

6. Remove it and repeat the process with the remaining tuna chaffle mixture.

7. Once ready, remove and enjoy warm.

Nutrition: **Calories**: 650 Cal; **Total Fat**: 39g; **Saturated Fat**: 0g; **Cholesterol**: 0mg; **Sodium**: 0mg; **Total Carbs**: 6g; **Fiber**: 0g; **Sugar**: 0g; **Protein**: 63g

160. GARLIC CHAFFLE STICKS

❤ **Servings:** 2

🧇 **Preparation Time**: 10 Minutes

⏰ **Cooking Time**: 15 Minutes

Ingredients:

- ✓ Two eggs
- ✓ 1 cup mozzarella cheese, grated
- ✓ 4 tablespoons almond flour
- ✓ 1 teaspoon garlic powder
- ✓ 1 teaspoon oregano
- ✓ ½ teaspoon salt

For the Topping:

- ✓ 4 tablespoons butter, unsalted softened
- ✓ ½ teaspoon garlic powder
- ✓ ½ cup mozzarella cheese, grated

Directions:

1. Preheat your waffle maker.

2. Whisk the eggs in a small bowl.

3. Add the almond flour, mozzarella, oregano, garlic powder, and salt. Mix well.

4. Spoon half of the egg mixture into your waffle maker. Cook for 5 minutes and remove it.

5. Repeat the process with the remaining batter and cook for 5 minutes.

6. Remove from the waffle maker and cut into four strips out of each waffle.

7. Place the waffle sticks on a tray and preheat your grill.

8. Add the butter and garlic powder to a small mixing bowl. Mix properly.

9. Using a brush, spread the garlic mixture over the sticks.

10. Sprinkle the shredded mozzarella over the sticks. Place under the grill for 3 minutes or until the cheese starts to melt and bubble.

11. Eat immediately!

Cheese is a significant ingredient when preparing chaffles. However, if you aren't a fan of cheese, there are many ways to get around it. Although they may not taste quite the same, almond milk ricotta is a delicious alternative to cheese! It has the consistency of contemporary cheese and provides a flavorful alternative to dairy cheese in many recipes.

Nutrition: **Calories**: 109; **Cal Total Fat**: 19g; **Saturated Fat**: 0g; **Cholesterol**: 0mg; **Sodium**: 0mg; **Total Carbs**: 7g; **Fiber**: 0g; **Sugar**: 0g; **Protein**: 27g

161. FRIED PICKLE CHAFFLE STICKS

♥ **Servings:** 1

▦ **Preparation Time:** 5 Minutes

⏰ **Cooking Time:** 15 Minutes

Ingredients:

- ✓ 1 egg
- ✓ 1/2 cup mozzarella cheese
- ✓ 1/4 cup pork panko
- ✓ 6-8 Pickle slices, thinly sliced
- ✓ 1 tablespoon pickle juice

Directions:

1. Mix all the ingredients, except the pickle slices, in a small bowl.

2. Use a paper towel to blot out excess liquid from the pickle slices.

3. Add a thin layer of the mixture to a preheated waffle iron.

4. Add some pickle slices before adding another thin layer of the mixture.

5. Close the waffle maker's lid and allow the mixture to cook for 4 minutes.

6. Optional: combine hot sauce with ranch to create a great-tasting dip.

Nutrition: **Calories:** 465 Cal; **Total Fat:** 22.7g; **Saturated Fat:** 0g; **Cholesterol:** 0mg; **Sodium:** 0mg; **Total Carbs:** 3.3g; **Fiber:** 0g; **Sugar:** 0g; **Protein:** 59.2g

162. SPICY JALAPENO POPPER CHAFFLES

♥ **Servings:** 1

▦ **Preparation Time:** 5 Minutes

⏰ **Cooking Time:** 10 Minutes

Ingredients: For the Chaffles:

- ✓ 1 egg
- ✓ 1 oz. Cream cheese softened
- ✓ 1 cup cheddar cheese, shredded

For the Topping:

- ✓ 2 tablespoons bacon bits
- ✓ 1/2 tablespoons jalapenos

Directions:

1. Turn on the waffle maker—preheat for up to 5 minutes.

2. Mix the chaffle Ingredients.

3. Pour the batter onto the waffle maker.

4. Cook the butter for 3-4 minutes until it's brown and crispy.

5. Sprinkle bacon bits and a few jalapeno slices as a topping.

Nutrition: **Calories:** 231 Cal; **Total Fat:** 18g; **Saturated Fat:** 0g; **Cholesterol:** 0mg; **Sodium:** 0mg; **Total Carbs:** 2g; **Fiber:** 0g; **Sugar:** 0g; **Protein:** 13g

163. EGGNOG CHAFFLES

💗 **Servings:** 1

🧇 **Preparation Time:** 5 Minutes

⏰ **Cooking Time:** 15 Minutes

Ingredients:

- ✓ 1 egg, separated
- ✓ 1 egg yolk
- ✓ 1/2 cup mozzarella cheese, shredded
- ✓ 1/2 teaspoon spiced rum
- ✓ 1 teaspoon vanilla extract
- ✓ 1/4 teaspoon nutmeg, dried
- ✓ A dash of cinnamon
- ✓ 1 teaspoon coconut flour

For the Icing:

- ✓ 2 tablespoons cream cheese
- ✓ 1 tablespoon powdered sweetener
- ✓ 2 teaspoons rum or rum extract

Directions:

1. Preheat the mini waffle maker.

2. Mix the egg yolk in a small bowl until smooth.

3. Add the coconut flour, cinnamon, and nutmeg. Mix well.

4. In another bowl, mix rum, egg white, and vanilla. Whisk until well combined.

5. Throw in the yolk mixture with the egg white mixture. You should be able to form a thin batter.

6. Add the mozzarella cheese and combine it with the mixture.

7. Separate the batter into two batches. Put 1/2 of the mixture into the waffle maker and let it cook for 6 minutes until it's reliable.

8. Repeat until you've used up the remaining batter.

9. In a separate bowl, mix all the icing ingredients.

10. Top the cooked chaffles with the icing, or you can use this as a dip.

Nutrition: Calories: 266 Cal; **Total Fat:** 23g

Saturated Fat: 0g; **Cholesterol:** 0mg; **Sodium:** 0mg; **Total Carbs:** 2g; **Fiber:** 0g; **Sugar:** 0g; **Protein:** 13g

164. KIMCHI CHEDDAR CHAFFLES

💗 **Servings:** 2

🧇 **Preparation Time:** 5 Minutes

⏰ **Cooking Time:** 35 Minutes

Ingredients:

- ✓ 2 cups of flour and cheddar cheese
- ✓ 1 cup cabbage Kimchi and buttermilk
- ✓ 1 teaspoon baking powder and soda
- ✓ Salt
- ✓ 1 teaspoon butter.
- ✓ 3 eggs
- ✓ 1 tablespoon chili peppers and scallion

Directions:

1. Heat the waffle maker and turn it on.

2. Combine baking powder, salt, and flour in a bowl.

3. In the next bowl, add Kimchi, cheese, eggs, buttermilk, butter, and scallion.

4. Pour the egg mix with the flour mix and place it on the waffle maker.

5. Cook it for 4 minutes and serve it with cream.

Nutrition: Calories: 676; **Carbohydrates:** 12g; **Protein:** 32g; **Fats:** 56g; **Saturated Fat:** 31g; **Fiber:** 6g; **Sugar:** 8g

165. RAISIN BELGIAN BREAD

Servings: 2

Preparation Time: 10 Minutes

Cooking Time: 10 Minutes

Ingredients:

- ✓ 1 cup almond flour
- ✓ 1 tablespoon baking powder and caraway seeds
- ✓ 1 cup of butter and almond milk
- ✓ 1 tablespoon Raisins, honey, sugar-free maple syrup, and oil
- ✓ 1 teaspoon baking powder and cinnamon
- ✓ 2 eggs

Directions:

1. Take one bowl and add almond flour to it. Stir it with few seeds, baking powder.

2. Add salt, cinnamon, and raisins to it. Take another bowl, add almond milk and eggs to it.

3. Put some butter and honey in it. Place it into the flour mix.

4. Pour the mixture into the maker and cook it for 4 minutes.

5. Serve it with sugar-free maple syrup.

Nutrition: Calories: 1291; **Carbohydrates:** 60g; **Protein:** 34g; **Fats:** 79g; **Saturated Fat:** 12.4g; **Fiber:** 30g; **Sugar:** 11g

166. KETO CHOCOLATE CHIP CHAFFLE

♥ **Servings:** 1

🧇 **Preparation Time:** 5 Minutes

⏰ **Cooking Time:** 8 Minutes

Ingredients:

- ✓ 1 egg
- ✓ 1/4 teaspoon baking powder
- ✓ A pinch of salt
- ✓ 1 tablespoon heavy whipping cream (topping)
- ✓ 1/2 teaspoon coconut flour
- ✓ 1 tablespoon Chocolate Chips
- ✓ 1 cup mozzarella cheese

Directions:

1. Preheat the mini waffle maker until hot.

2. Whisk the egg in a bowl, add the cheese, and then mix well.

3. Stir in the remaining ingredients (except toppings, if any).

4. Grease the preheated waffle maker. This will help to create a crisper crust.

5. Scoop 1/2 of the batter onto the waffle maker, spread across evenly.

6. Sprinkle chocolate chips on top.

7. Cook until a bit browned and crispy, about 4 minutes.

8. Gently remove from the waffle maker and let it cool.

9. Repeat with the remaining batter.

10. Top with whipping cream.

11. Serve and Enjoy!

Nutrition: **Calories:** 110; **Carbs:** 16g; **Protein:** 6g; **Fats:** 4g; **Phosphorus:** 138mg; **Potassium:** 745mg; **Sodium:** 214mg

167. CHOCOLATE CHIP CANNOLI CHAFFLES

♥ **Servings:** 2

🧇 **Preparation Time:** 15 Minutes

⏰ **Cooking Time:** 5 Minutes

Ingredients: For the Chocolate Chip Chaffle:

- ✓ 1 tablespoon. butter, melted
- ✓ 1 tablespoon. monk fruit
- ✓ 1 egg yolk
- ✓ 1/8 teaspoon vanilla extract
- ✓ 3 tablespoon. almond flour
- ✓ 1/8 teaspoon baking powder
- ✓ 1 tablespoon. chocolate chips, sugar-free

For the Cannoli Topping:

- ✓ 2 oz. Cream cheese
- ✓ 2 tablespoon. low-carb confectioners' sweetener
- ✓ 6 tablespoon. ricotta cheese, full fat
- ✓ 1/4 teaspoon vanilla extract
- ✓ 5 Drops lemon extract

Directions:

1. Preheat the mini waffle maker.

2. Mix all the ingredients for the chocolate chip chaffle in a mixing bowl. Combine well to make a batter.

3. Place half the batter on the waffle maker. Allow to cooking for 3-4 minutes.

4. While waiting for the chaffles to cooking, start making your cannoli topping by combining all ingredients until the consistency is creamy and smooth.

5. Place the cannoli topping on the cooked chaffles before serving.

Nutrition: **Calories**: 123; **Carbs**: 16.5g; **Protein**: 2g; **Fats**: 6g; **Phosphorus**: 56mg; **Potassium**: 450mg; **Sodium**: 35mg

168. OREO CHAFFLE

Servings: 2

Preparation Time: 10 Minutes

Cooking Time: 20 Minutes

Ingredients:

- ✓ 2 teaspoons coconut flour
- ✓ 3 tablespoons cocoa, unsweetened
- ✓ 1 teaspoon baking powder
- ✓ 4 tablespoons swerve sweetener
- ✓ 1 teaspoon vanilla extract, unsweetened
- ✓ 2 tablespoons heavy cream
- ✓ 2 eggs, at room temperature
- ✓ 2 tablespoons whipped cream

Directions:

1. Take a non-stick waffle iron, plug it in, select the medium or medium-high heat setting and let it preheat until ready to use; it could also be indicated with an indicator light changing its color.

2. Meanwhile, mix the batter and for this, take a large bowl, add flour in it along with other ingredients and mix with an electric mixer until smooth.

3. Use a ladle to pour a quarter of the prepared batter into the heated waffle iron in a spiral direction, starting from the edges, then shut the lid and cook for 5 minutes or more until solid and nicely browned; the cooked waffle will look like a cake.

4. When done, transfer chaffles to a plate with a silicone spatula and repeat with the remaining batter.

5. When done, prepare the Oreo sandwiches, and for this, spread 1 tablespoon of whipped cream on one side of two chaffles and then cover with the remaining chaffles.

6. Serve immediately.

Nutrition: **Calories**: 295.6; **Fats**: 18.7g; **Carbs**: 11g; **Fiber**: 2.2g; **Potassium**: 140mg; **Sodium**: 6.8mg; **Phosphorous**:58g; **Protein**: 20.7g

169. KETO ICE CREAM CHAFFLE

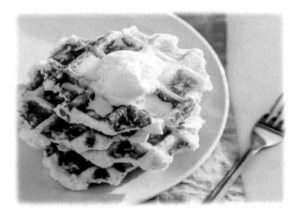

♥ **Servings:** 2

▦ **Preparation Time**: 15 Minutes

⏰ **Cooking Time**: 30 Minutes

Ingredients:

- ✓ 1 egg
- ✓ 2 tablespoons Swerve/Monk fruit
- ✓ 1 tablespoon Baking powder
- ✓ 1 tablespoon Heavy whipping cream
- ✓ Keto ice cream, as desired

Directions:

1. Take a small bowl and whisk the egg and add all the ingredients.

2. Beat until the mixture becomes creamy.

3. Pour the mixture into the lower plate of the waffle maker and spread it evenly to cover the plate properly.

4. Close the lid.

5. Cook for at least 4 minutes to get the desired crunch.

6. Remove the chaffle from the heat and keep it aside for a few minutes.

7. Make as many chaffles as your mixture and waffle maker allow.

8. Top with your favorite ice cream, and enjoy!

> **Nutrition:** **Calories:** 88; **Fat:** 1g; **Carbohydrates:** 19g; **Phosphorus:** 74mg; **Potassium**: 92mg; **Sodium:** 47mg; **Protein:** 1g

170. MOZZARELLA LEMONY CHAFFLES

♥ **Servings:** 2

▦ **Preparation Time**: 5 Minutes

⏰ **Cooking Time**: 17 Minutes

Ingredients:

- ✓ 2 eggs
- ✓ 1 cup Shredded mozzarella
- ✓ 2 tablespoons Lemon juice
- ✓ 2 teaspoons Any keto sweetener
- ✓ 2 teaspoons Coconut flour

Directions:

1. Preheat your mini waffle iron if needed and grease it.

2. Mix all the ingredients in a bowl and whisk.

3. Cook your mixture in the mini waffle iron for at least 4 minutes.

4. Serve hot and make as many chaffles as your mixture and waffle maker allow.

Nutrition: **Calories**: 165; **Fat**: 2g; **Carbohydrates**: 2g; **Protein**: 26g

171. DOUBLE CHOCOLATE CHAFFLE

♥ **Servings**: 2

Preparation Time: 5 Minutes

Cooking Time: 10 Minutes

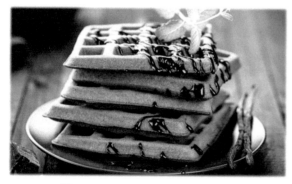

Ingredients:

- ✓ 2 eggs
- ✓ 4 tablespoons Coconut flour
- ✓ 2 tablespoons Cocoa powder
- ✓ 2 oz. Cream cheese
- ✓ ½ teaspoon Baking powder
- ✓ 2 tablespoons (unsweetened) Chocolate chips
- ✓ 1 teaspoon Vanilla extract
- ✓ 4 tablespoons Swerve/Monk fruit

Directions:

1. Preheat a mini waffle maker if needed and grease it.

2. In a mixing bowl, beat the eggs.

3. In a separate mixing bowl, add coconut flour, cocoa powder, Swerve/Monk fruit, and baking powder; when combined, pour into the eggs with cream cheese and vanilla extracts.

4. Mix them all well to give them uniform consistency, and pour the mixture to the lower plate of the waffle maker.

5. On top of the mixture, sprinkle a half teaspoon of unsweetened chocolate chips around and close the lid.

6. Cook for at least 4 minutes to get the desired crunch.

7. Remove the chaffle from the heat and keep it aside for around one minute.

8. Make as many chaffles as your mixture and waffle maker allow.

9. Serve with your favorite whipped cream or berries.

Nutrition: **Calories**: 87; **Fat**: 1g; **Carbohydrates**: 22g; **Phosphorus**: 28mg; **Potassium**: 192mg; **Sodium**: 3mg; **Protein**: 1g

172. CREAM CHEESE MINI CHAFFLE

💔 **Servings:** 2

🍞 **Preparation Time:** 5 Minutes

⏰ **Cooking Time:** 10 Minutes

Ingredients:

- ✓ 1 egg
- ✓ 2 tablespoons Coconut flour
- ✓ 1 oz. Cream cheese
- ✓ ¼ teaspoon Baking powder
- ✓ ½ teaspoon Vanilla extract
- ✓ 4 teaspoons Swerve/Monk fruit

Directions:

1. Preheat a waffle maker and grease it if needed.

2. In a mixing bowl, mix coconut flour, Swerve/Monk fruit, and baking powder.

3. Now add the egg to the mixture with cream cheese and vanilla extract.

4. Mix them all well and pour the mixture to the lower plate of the waffle maker.

5. Close the lid.

6. Cook for at least 4 minutes to get the desired crunch.

7. Remove the chaffle from the heat.

8. Make as many chaffles as your mixture and waffle maker allow.

9. Eat the chaffles with your favorite toppings.

> **Nutrition: Calories:** 47; **Fat:** 0g; **Carbohydrates:** 11g; **Phosphorus:** 30mg; **Potassium:** 197mg; **Sodium:** 4mg; **Protein:** 1g

173. BLACKBERRIES CHAFFLE

💔 **Servings:** 2

🍞 **Preparation Time:** 15 Minutes

⏰ **Cooking Time:** 20 Minutes

Ingredients:

- ✓ 1/3 cup Cheddar cheese
- ✓ 1 egg
- ✓ 1/2 cup Blackberries
- ✓ 2 tablespoons Almond flour
- ✓ 1/4 teaspoon Baking powder
- ✓ 2 tablespoons ground almonds
- ✓ 1/3 cup mozzarella cheese

Directions:

1. Mix cheddar cheese, egg, blackberries, almond flour, almond ground, and baking powder together in a bowl.

2. Preheat your waffle iron and grease it.

3. In your mini waffle iron, shred half of the Mozzarella cheese.

4. Add the mixture to your mini waffle iron.

5. Again, shred the remaining mozzarella cheese on the mixture.

6. Cook till the desired crisp is achieved.

7. Make as many chaffles as your mixture and waffle maker allow.

Nutrition: **Calories:** 243; **Fat:** 11g; **Carbohydrates:** 33g; **Phosphorus:** 84mg; **Potassium:** 189mg; **Sodium:** 145mg; **Protein:** 4g

174. CHOCO CHIP CANNOLI CHAFFLE

Servings: 2

Preparation Time: 10 Minutes

Cooking Time: 20 Minutes

Ingredients: For the Chaffle:

- ✓ 1 egg yolk
- ✓ 1 tablespoon Swerve/Monk fruit
- ✓ 1/8 tablespoon Baking powder
- ✓ 1/8 teaspoon Vanilla extract
- ✓ 3 tablespoons Almond flour
- ✓ 1 tablespoon Chocolate chips

For the Cannoli Topping:

- ✓ 4 tablespoons Cream cheese
- ✓ 6 tablespoons Ricotta
- ✓ 2 tablespoons Sweetener
- ✓ ¼ tablespoon Vanilla extract
- ✓ 5 Drops Lemon extract

Directions:

1. Preheat a mini waffle maker and grease it if needed.

2. In a mixing bowl, add all the chaffle ingredients and mix well.

3. Pour the mixture to the lower plate of the waffle maker and spread it evenly to cover the plate properly, and close the lid.

4. Cook for at least 4 minutes to get the desired crunch.

5. In the meanwhile, prepare the cannoli topping by adding all the ingredients to the blender to give the creamy texture.

6. Remove the chaffle from the heat and keep it aside to cool it down.

7. Make as many chaffles as your mixture and waffle maker allow.

8. Serve with the cannoli toppings and enjoy.

Nutrition: **Calories:** 159; **Fat:** 1g **Carbohydrates:** 34g; **Phosphorus** 130mg; **Potassium:** 116mg; **Sodium:** 33mg; **Protein:** 4g

175. TOMATO ONIONS CHAFFLES

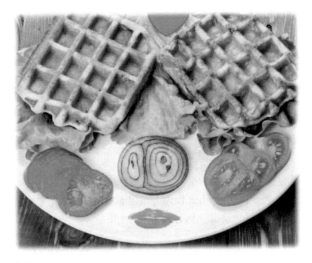

💗 **Servings:** 2

🧇 **Preparation Time:** 10 Minutes

⏰ **Cooking Time:** 20 Minutes

Ingredients: For the Chaffle:

- ✓ 1 egg
- ✓ 1/2 cup Mozzarella cheese (shredded)
- ✓ ½ cup chopped onion
- ✓ ½ teaspoon garlic powder
- ✓ ½ teaspoon Dried basil

For the Topping:

- ✓ 1 Large thickly sliced tomato
- ✓ ½ cup (shredded) mozzarella cheese
- ✓ ½ teaspoon oregano

Directions:

1. Preheat a mini waffle maker if needed and grease it.

2. In a mixing bowl, add all the ingredients of the chaffle and mix well.

3. Pour the mixture into the waffle maker.

4. Cook for at least 4 minutes to get the desired crunch, and make as many chaffles as your batter allows.

5. Preheat the oven.

6. Spread the chaffles on the baking sheet and top with one tomato slice.

7. Sprinkle cheese on top and put the baking sheet into the oven.

8. Heat for 5 minutes to melt the cheese.

9. Spread oregano on top and serve hot.

Nutrition: **Calories:** 175; **Fat:** 10g

Carbohydrates: 19g; **Phosphorus:** 111mg

Potassium: 170mg; **Sodium:** 62mg; **Protein:** 5g

133

176. CREAM CHEESE PUMPKIN CHAFFLE

💜 **Servings:** 2

🧇 **Preparation Time**: 5 Minutes

⏰ **Cooking Time**: 10 Minutes

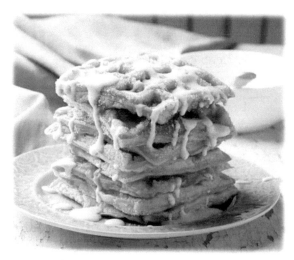

Ingredients:

- ✓ 2 eggs
- ✓ 2 oz. Cream cheese
- ✓ 2 teaspoons Coconut flour
- ✓ 4 teaspoons Swerve/Monk fruit
- ✓ ½ teaspoon Baking powder
- ✓ 1 teaspoon Vanilla extract
- ✓ 2 tablespoons canned pumpkin
- ✓ ½ teaspoon Pumpkin spice

Directions:

1. Take a small mixing bowl and add Swerve/Monk fruit, coconut flour, and baking powder and mix them all well.

2. Now add the egg, vanilla extract, pumpkin, and cream cheese, and beat them all together till uniform consistency is achieved.

3. Preheat a mini waffle maker if needed.

4. Pour the mixture into the greasy waffle maker.

5. Cook for at least 4 minutes to get the desired crunch.

6. Remove the chaffle from the heat.

7. Make as many chaffles as your mixture and waffle maker allow

8. Serve with butter or whipped cream that you like!

Nutrition: **Calories**: 197; **Fat**: 4g

Carbohydrates: 35g; **Phosphorus**: 109mg

Potassium: 192mg; **Sodium**: 159mg; **Protein**: 6g

177. BERRIES-COCONUT CHAFFLES

💜 **Servings:** 2

🧇 **Preparation Time**: 5 Minutes

⏰ **Cooking Time**: 20 Minutes

Ingredients:

- ✓ 1/3 cup Cheddar cheese
- ✓ 1 egg
- ✓ ½ cup Blackberries
- ✓ 2 tablespoons Coconut flour
- ✓ 1/4 teaspoon Baking powder
- ✓ 2 tablespoons coconut flakes
- ✓ 1/3 cup mozzarella cheese

Directions:

1. Mix cheddar cheese, egg, coconut flour, coconut flakes, blackberries, and baking powder together in a bowl

2. Preheat your waffle iron and grease it.

3. In your mini waffle iron, shred half of the mozzarella cheese.

4. Add the mixture to your mini waffle iron.

5. Again, shred the remaining mozzarella cheese on the mixture.

6. Cook till the desired crisp is achieved.

7. Make as many chaffles as your mixture and waffle maker allow.

Nutrition: Calories: 331; **Fat**: 11g

Carbohydrates: 52g; **Phosphorus**: 90mg

Potassium: 89mg; **Sodium**: 35mg; **Protein**: 6g

178. PLUM AND ALMONDS CHAFFLE

💗 **Servings:** 2

🪨 **Preparation Time**: 15 Minutes

⏰ **Cooking Time**: 20 Minutes

Ingredients:

- ✓ 1/3 cup cheddar cheese
- ✓ 1 egg
- ✓ 1 tablespoon lemon juice
- ✓ ½ cup puree plum
- ✓ 2 tablespoons almond flour
- ✓ 1/4 teaspoon baking powder
- ✓ 2 tablespoons ground almonds
- ✓ 1/3 cup mozzarella cheese

Directions:

1. Mix cheddar cheese, egg, lemon juice, almond flour, plum, almond ground, and baking powder together in a bowl.

2. Preheat your waffle iron and grease it.

3. In your mini waffle iron, shred half of the mozzarella cheese.

4. Add the mixture to your mini waffle iron.

5. Again, shred the remaining mozzarella cheese on the mixture.

6. Cook till the desired crisp is achieved.

7. Make as many chaffles as your mixture and waffle maker allow.

179. EASY BLUEBERRY CHAFFLE

Servings: 2

Preparation Time: 5 Minutes

Cooking Time: 10 Minutes

Ingredients:

- ✓ 2 eggs
- ✓ 2 oz. Cream cheese
- ✓ 2 tablespoons coconut flour
- ✓ 4 teaspoons Swerve/Monk fruit:
- ✓ ½ teaspoon baking powder
- ✓ 1 teaspoon vanilla extract
- ✓ ½ cup blueberries

Directions:

1. Take a small mixing bowl and add Swerve/Monk fruit, baking powder, and coconut flour and mix them all well.

2. Now add the eggs, vanilla extract, and cream cheese, and beat them all together till uniform consistency is achieved.

3. Preheat a mini waffle maker and grease it if needed.

4. Pour the mixture into the lower plate of the waffle maker.

5. Add 3-4 fresh blueberries above the mixture and close the lid.

6. Cook for at least 4 minutes to get the desired crunch.

7. Remove the chaffle from the heat.

8. Make as many chaffles as your mixture and waffle maker allow.

9. Serve with butter or whipped cream that you like!

Nutrition: Calories: 304; **Fat**: 29g

Carbohydrates: 12g; **Phosphorus**: 119mg

Potassium: 109mg; **Sodium**: 204mg; **Protein**: 9g

180. ZUCCHINI CHAFFLE

A nice and refreshing way to eat your chaffle. Ready in no time, perfect for snack or dinner.

💙 **Servings**: 2

🍳 **Preparation Time**: 5 Minutes

⏰ **Cooking Time**: 15 Minutes

Ingredients: For the Batter:

- ✓ 4 eggs
- ✓ 1 cup grated mozzarella cheese
- ✓ 1 cup grated pepper jack cheese
- ✓ 1 small zucchini, grated
- ✓ 3 tablespoons almond flour
- ✓ 2 tablespoons coconut flour
- ✓ 2½ teaspoons baking powder
- ✓ Salt and pepper to taste

Other:

- ✓ 2 tablespoons butter to brush the waffle maker

Directions:

1. Preheat the waffle maker.
2. Add the eggs, cheeses, zucchini, almond flour, coconut flour, baking powder, and salt and pepper to a bowl.
3. Mix with a fork.
4. Brush the heated waffle maker with butter and add a few tablespoons of the batter.
5. Close the lid and cook for about 5–7 minutes, depending on your waffle maker.
6. Serve and enjoy.

Nutrition: **Calories**: 298; **Fat**: 23.3g; **Carbs**: 6.7g; **Sugar**: 0.9g; **Protein**: 16.6g; **Sodium**: 323mg

181. MUSHROOM AND ALMOND CHAFFLE

A delicious and crunchy chaffle is always a good idea. Stay healthy and eat clean while on the keto diet.

Servings: 2

Preparation Time: 5 Minutes

Cooking Time: 15 Minutes

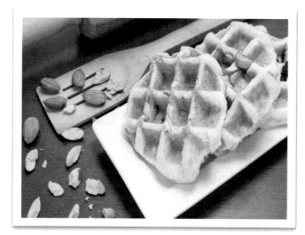

Ingredients: For the Batter:

- ✓ 4 eggs
- ✓ 2 cups grated mozzarella cheese
- ✓ 1 cup finely chopped zucchini
- ✓ 3 tablespoons chopped almonds
- ✓ 2 teaspoons baking powder
- ✓ Salt and pepper to taste
- ✓ 1 teaspoon dried basil
- ✓ 1 teaspoon chili flakes

Other:

- ✓ 2 tablespoons cooking spray to brush the waffle maker

Directions:

1. Preheat the waffle maker.

2. Add the eggs, grated mozzarella, mushrooms, almonds, baking powder, salt and pepper, dried basil, and chili flakes to a bowl.

3. Mix with a fork.

4. Brush the heated waffle maker with cooking spray and add a few tablespoons of the batter.

5. Close the lid and cook for about 5–7 minutes, depending on your waffle maker.

6. Serve and enjoy.

Nutrition: **Calories**: 196; **Fat**: 16g; **Carbs**: 4g; **Sugar**: 1g; **Protein**: 10.8g; **Sodium**: 152mg

182. AVOCADO CROQUE MADAM CHAFFLE

A nice French classic, transformed into a keto-friendly option. Who doesn't love a nice Croque Madam?

❤ **Servings: 2**

▨ **Preparation Time: 5 Minutes**

⏰ **Cooking Time: 15 Minutes**

Ingredients: Fort the Batter:

- ✓ 4 eggs
- ✓ 2 cups grated mozzarella cheese
- ✓ 1 Avocado, mashed
- ✓ Salt and pepper to taste
- ✓ 6 tablespoons almond flour
- ✓ 2 teaspoons baking powder
- ✓ 1 teaspoon dried dill

Other:

- ✓ 2 tablespoons cooking spray to brush the waffle maker
- ✓ 4 Fried eggs
- ✓ 2 tablespoons freshly chopped basil

Directions:

1. Preheat the waffle maker.

2. Add the eggs, grated mozzarella, avocado, salt and pepper, almond flour, baking powder, and dried dill to a bowl.

3. Mix with a fork.

4. Brush the heated waffle maker with cooking spray and add a few tablespoons of the batter.

5. Close the lid and cook for about 5–7 minutes, depending on your waffle maker.

6. Serve each chaffle with a fried egg and freshly chopped basil on top.

> **Nutrition: Calories:** 393; **Fat:** 32.1g; **Carbs:** 9.2g; **Sugar:** 1.3g; **Protein:** 18.8g; **Sodium:** 245mg

183. SPINACH AND ARTICHOKE CHAFFLE

A nice spinach chaffle is always a good idea to eat well during your keto diet.

❤ **Servings:** 2

▨ **Preparation Time:** 5 Minutes

⏰ **Cooking Time:** 15 Minutes

Ingredients: For the Batter:

- ✓ 4 eggs
- ✓ 2 cups grated provolone cheese
- ✓ 1 cup cooked and diced spinach
- ✓ ½ cup diced artichoke hearts
- ✓ Salt and pepper to taste
- ✓ 2 tablespoons coconut flour
- ✓ 2 teaspoons baking powder

Other:

- ✓ 2 tablespoons cooking spray to brush the waffle maker
- ✓ ¼ cup of cream cheese for serving

Directions:

1. Preheat the waffle maker.

2. Add the eggs, grated provolone cheese, diced spinach, artichoke hearts, salt and pepper, coconut flour, and baking powder to a bowl.

3. Mix with a fork.

4. Brush the heated waffle maker with cooking spray and add a few tablespoons of the batter.

5. Close the lid and cook for about 5–7 minutes, depending on your waffle maker.

6. Serve each chaffle with cream cheese.

Nutrition: Calories: 427; **Fat:** 32.8g; **Carbs:** 9.5g; **Sugar:** 1.1g; **Protein:** 25.7g; **Sodium:** 722mg

184. ASPARAGUS CHAFFLE

Are you looking for a new way of eating your asparagus? Here is an incredible recipe.

❤ **Servings:** 2

▨ **Preparation Time:** 5 Minutes

⏰ **Cooking Time:** 15 Minutes

Ingredients: For the Batter:

- ✓ 4 eggs
- ✓ 1½ cups grated mozzarella cheese
- ✓ ½ cup grated parmesan cheese
- ✓ 1 cup boiled asparagus, chopped
- ✓ Salt and pepper to taste
- ✓ ¼ cup almond flour
- ✓ 2 teaspoons baking powder

Other:

- ✓ 2 tablespoons cooking spray to brush the waffle maker
- ✓ ¼ cup Greek yogurt for serving
- ✓ ¼ cup chopped almonds for serving

Directions:

1. Preheat the waffle maker.

2. Add the eggs, grated mozzarella, grated parmesan, asparagus, salt and pepper, almond flour, and baking powder to a bowl.

3. Mix with a fork.

4. Brush the heated waffle maker with cooking spray and add a few tablespoons of the batter.

5. Close the lid and cook for about 5–7 minutes, depending on your waffle maker.

6. Serve each chaffle with Greek yogurt and chopped almonds.

Nutrition: **Calories:** 316; **Fat:** 24.9g; **Carbs:** 7.3g;**Sugar:** 1.2g; **Protein:** 18.2g; **Sodium:** 261mg

185. BROCCOLI CHAFFLE

Even if you are not such a fan of broccoli, you are going to love this recipe.

Servings: 2

Preparation Time: 5 Minutes

Cooking Time: 15 Minutes

Ingredients: For the Batter:

- ✓ 4 eggs
- ✓ 2 cups grated mozzarella cheese
- ✓ 1 cup steamed broccoli, chopped
- ✓ Salt and pepper to taste
- ✓ 1 Clove garlic, minced
- ✓ 1 teaspoon chili flakes
- ✓ 2 tablespoons almond flour
- ✓ 2 teaspoons baking powder

Other:

- ✓ 2 tablespoons cooking spray to brush the waffle maker
- ✓ ¼ cup mascarpone cheese for serving

Directions:

1. Preheat the waffle maker.

2. Add the eggs, grated mozzarella, chopped broccoli, salt and pepper, minced garlic, chili flakes, almond flour, and baking powder to a bowl.

3. Mix with a fork.

4. Brush the heated waffle maker with cooking spray and add a few tablespoons of the batter.

5. Close the lid and cook for about 5–7 minutes, depending on your waffle maker.

6. Serve each chaffle with mascarpone cheese.

Nutrition: **Calories:** 229; **Fat:** 17.5g; **Carbs:** 6g; **Sugar:** 1.1g; **Protein:** 13.1g; **Sodium:** 194mg

186. CAULIFLOWER CHAFFLE

This recipe is one of the best ways to use cauliflower. An unforgettable chaffle experience.

❤ **Servings**: 2

▦ **Preparation Time**: 5 Minutes

⏰ **Cooking Time**: 15 Minutes

Ingredients: For the Batter:

- ✓ 4 eggs
- ✓ 2 cups grated cheddar cheese
- ✓ 1 cup steamed cauliflower, chopped
- ✓ Salt and pepper to taste
- ✓ 1 teaspoon dried basil
- ✓ ½ teaspoon onion powder
- ✓ 2 tablespoons almond flour
- ✓ 2 teaspoons baking powder

Other:

- ✓ 2 tablespoons cooking spray to brush the waffle maker
- ✓ ¼ cup mascarpone cheese for serving

Directions:

1. Preheat the waffle maker.

2. Add the eggs, grated cheddar, cauliflower, salt and pepper, dried basil, onion powder, almond flour, and baking powder to a bowl.

3. Mix with a fork.

4. Brush the heated waffle maker with cooking spray and add a few tablespoons of the batter.

5. Close the lid and cook for about 5–7 minutes, depending on your waffle maker.

6. Serve each chaffle with mascarpone cheese.

Nutrition: **Calories**: 409; **Fat**: 33.7g; **Carbs**: 5g; **Sugar**: 1.4g; **Protein**: 22.7g; **Sodium**: 434mg

187. CELERY AND COTTAGE CHEESE CHAFFLE

This is a flavor combination made in heaven. Everyone will love this chaffle recipe.

❤ **Servings**: 2

▦ **Preparation Time**: 5 Minutes

⏰ **Cooking Time**: 15 Minutes

Ingredients: For the Batter:

- ✓ 4 eggs
- ✓ 2 cups grated cheddar cheese
- ✓ 1 cup fresh celery, chopped
- ✓ Salt and pepper to taste
- ✓ 2 tablespoons chopped almonds
- ✓ 2 teaspoons baking powder

Other:

- ✓ 2 tablespoons cooking spray to brush the waffle maker
- ✓ ¼ cup cottage cheese for serving

Directions:

1. Preheat the waffle maker.

2. Add the eggs, grated mozzarella cheese, chopped celery, salt and pepper, chopped almonds, and baking powder to a bowl.

3. Mix with a fork.

4. Brush the heated waffle maker with cooking spray and add a few tablespoons of the batter.

5. Close the lid and cook for about 5–7 minutes, depending on your waffle maker.

6. Serve each chaffle with cottage cheese on top.

Nutrition: **Calories**: 385; **Fat**: 31.6g; **Carbs**: 4g; **Sugar**: 1.5g; **Protein**: 22.2g; **Sodium**: 492mg

188. CRISPY BAGEL CHAFFLES

♥ **Servings:** 2

🧇 **Preparation Time**: 5 Minutes

⏰ **Cooking Time**: 30 Minutes

Ingredients:

- ✓ 2 eggs
- ✓ ½ cup parmesan cheese
- ✓ 1 teaspoon bagel seasoning
- ✓ ½ cup mozzarella cheese
- ✓ 2 teaspoons almond flour

Directions:

1. Turn on the waffle maker to heat and oil it with cooking spray.

2. Evenly sprinkle half of the cheeses to a griddle and let them melt. Then toast for 30 seconds and leave them to wait for the batter.

3. Whisk eggs, the other half of cheeses, almond flour, and bagel seasoning in a small bowl.

4. Pour some batter into the waffle maker—cook for 4-5 minutes.

5. Let cool for 2-3 minutes before serving.

Nutrition: **Calories**: 117; **Fat**: 2.1g; **Carbs**: 18.2g; **Protein**: 22.7g; **Potassium**: (K) 296mg**Sodium**: (Na) 81mg; **Phosphorous**: 28mg

189. BROCCOLI & ALMOND FLOUR CHAFFLES

💗 **Servings:** 2

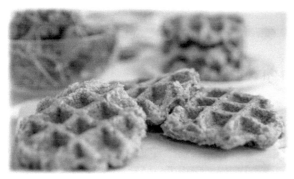

🧇 **Preparation Time:** 6 Minutes

⏰ **Cooking Time:** 8 Minutes

Ingredients:

- ✓ 1 Organic egg, beaten
- ✓ ½ cup Cheddar cheese, shredded
- ✓ ¼ cup fresh broccoli, chopped
- ✓ 1 tablespoon almond flour
- ✓ ¼ teaspoon garlic powder

Directions:

1. Preheat a mini waffle maker and then grease it.

2. In a bowl, place all ingredients and mix until well combined.

3. Place half of the mixture into the preheated waffle iron and cook for about four minutes or until golden brown.

4. Repeat with the remaining mixture.

5. Serve warm.

Nutrition: **Calories:** 221; **Protein:** 17g

Carbs: 31g; **Fat:** 8g; **Sodium:** (Na) 235mg

Potassium: (K) 176mg; **Phosphorus:** 189mg

---

190. CHEDDAR JALAPEÑO CHAFFLE

💗 **Servings:** 2

🧇 **Preparation Time:** 6 Minutes

⏰ **Cooking Time:** 5 Minutes

Ingredients:

- ✓ 2 large eggs
- ✓ ½ cup shredded mozzarella
- ✓ ¼ cup almond flour
- ✓ ½ teaspoon baking powder
- ✓ ¼ cup shredded cheddar cheese
- ✓ 2 tablespoons diced jalapeños jarred or canned

For the Toppings:

- ✓ ½ Cooked bacon, chopped
- ✓ 2 tablespoons cream cheese
- ✓ ¼ Jalapeño slices

Directions:

1. Turn on the waffle maker to heat and oil it with cooking spray.

2. Mix the mozzarella, eggs, baking powder, almond flour, and garlic powder in a bowl.

3. Sprinkle two tablespoons cheddar cheese in a thin layer on the waffle maker, and ½ jalapeño.

4. Ladle half of the egg mixture on top of the cheese and jalapeños.

5. Cook for 4-5 minutes, or until done.

6. Repeat for the second chaffle.

7. Top with cream cheese, bacon, and jalapeño slices.

Nutrition: **Calories:** 221; **Protein:** 13g; **Carbs:** 1g; **Fat:** 34g; **Sodium:** (Na) 80mg; **Potassium:** (K) 119mg; **Phosphorus:** 158mg

191. TACO CHAFFLES

❤ **Servings:** 2

Preparation Time: 10 Minutes

⏰ **Cooking Time:** 20 Minutes

Ingredients:

- ✓ 1 tablespoon almond flour
- ✓ 1 cup taco blend cheese
- ✓ 2 organic eggs
- ✓ ¼ teaspoon taco seasoning

Directions:

1. Preheat a mini waffle maker and then grease it.

2. In a bowl, place all ingredients and mix until well combined.

3. Place ¼ of the mixture into the preheated waffle iron and cook for about four minutes or until golden brown.

4. Repeat with the remaining mixture.

5. Serve warm.

Nutrition: **Calories:** 221; **Protein:** 14g; **Carbs:** 3g; **Fat:** 2g; **Sodium:** (Na) 119mg; **Potassium:** (K) 398mg; **Phosphorus:** 149mg

192. SPINACH & CAULIFLOWER CHAFFLES

❤ **Servings:** 2

🍴 **Preparation Time:** 6 Minutes

⏰ **Cooking Time:** 10 Minutes

Ingredients:

- ✓ ½ cup frozen chopped spinach, thawed and squeezed
- ✓ ½ cup cauliflower, chopped finely
- ✓ ½ cup Cheddar cheese, shredded
- ✓ ½ cup Mozzarella cheese, shredded
- ✓ 1/3 cup Parmesan cheese, shredded
- ✓ 2 organic eggs
- ✓ 1 tablespoon butter, melted
- ✓ 1 teaspoon garlic powder
- ✓ 1 teaspoon onion powder
- ✓ Salt and freshly ground black pepper, to taste

Directions:

1. Preheat a waffle iron and then grease it.

2. In a medium bowl, place all ingredients and mix until well combined.

3. Place half of the mixture into the preheated waffle iron and cook for about 4-5 minutes or until golden brown.

4. Repeat with the remaining mixture.

5. Serve warm.

Nutrition: **Calories:** 221; **Protein:** 11g; **Carbs:** 26g; **Fat:** 7g; **Sodium:** (Na) 143mg; **Potassium:** (K)197mg; **Phosphorus:** 182mg

193. ROSEMARY IN CHAFFLES

❤ **Servings:** 2

🍴 **Preparation Time:** 6 Minutes

⏰ **Cooking Time:** 8 Minutes

Ingredients:

- ✓ 1 organic egg, beaten
- ✓ ½ cup Cheddar cheese, shredded
- ✓ 1 tablespoon almond flour
- ✓ 1 tablespoon fresh rosemary, chopped
- ✓ A pinch of salt and freshly ground black pepper

Directions:

1. Preheat a mini waffle maker and then grease it.

2. For the chaffles, in a medium bowl, place all ingredients and with a fork, mix until well combined.

3. Place half of the mixture into the preheated waffle iron and cook for about four minutes or until golden brown.

4. Repeat with the remaining mixture.

5. Serve warm.

Nutrition: **Calories:** 221; **Protein:** 12g; **Carbs:** 29g; **Fat:** 8g; **Sodium:** (Na) 398mg; **Potassium:** (K) 347mg; **Phosphorus:** 241mg

194. ZUCCHINI IN CHAFFLES

❤ **Servings:** 2

🧇 **Preparation Time**: 10 Minutes

⏰ **Cooking Time**: 18 Minutes

Ingredients:

- ✓ 2 large zucchinis, grated and squeezed
- ✓ 2 large organic eggs
- ✓ 2/3 cup Cheddar cheese, shredded
- ✓ 2 tablespoons coconut flour
- ✓ ½ teaspoon garlic powder
- ✓ ½ teaspoon red pepper flakes, crushed
- ✓ Salt, to taste

Directions:

1. Preheat a waffle iron and then grease it.

2. In a medium bowl, place all ingredients and mix until well combined.

3. Place ¼ of the mixture into the preheated waffle iron and cook for about 4-4½ minutes or until golden brown.

4. Repeat with the remaining mixture.

5. Serve warm.

Nutrition: **Calories:** 311; **Protein:** 16g; **Carbs:** 17g; **Fat:** 15g; **Sodium:** (Na) 31mg; **Potassium:** (K) 418mg; **Phosphorus:** 257mg

195. 3-CHEESE BROCCOLI CHAFFLES

♥ **Servings:** 2

▦ **Preparation Time:** 10 Minutes

⏰ **Cooking Time:** 16 Minutes

Ingredients:

- ½ cup cooked broccoli, chopped finely
- 2 organic eggs, beaten
- ½ cup Cheddar cheese, shredded
- ½ cup Mozzarella cheese, shredded
- 2 tablespoons Parmesan cheese, grated
- ½ teaspoon onion powder

Directions:

1. Preheat a waffle iron and then grease it.

2. In a bowl, place all ingredients and mix until well combined.

3. Place half of the mixture into the preheated waffle iron and cook for about four minutes or until golden brown.

4. Repeat with the remaining mixture.

5. Serve warm.

Nutrition: **Calories:** 199; **Protein:** 19g

Carbs: 7g; **Fat:** 8g; **Sodium:** (Na) 466mg

Potassium: (K) 251mg; **Phosphorus:** 211mg

196. GARLIC AND ONION POWDER CHAFFLES

♥ **Servings:** 2

▦ **Preparation Time:** 5 Minutes

⏰ **Cooking Time:** 5 Minutes

Ingredients:

- 1 organic egg, beaten
- ¼ cup Cheddar cheese, shredded
- 2 tablespoons almond flour
- ½ teaspoon organic baking powder
- ¼ teaspoon garlic powder
- ¼ teaspoon onion powder
- A pinch of salt

Directions:

1. Preheat a waffle iron and then grease it.

2. In a bowl, place all the ingredients and beat until well combined.

3. Place the mixture into the preheated waffle iron and cook for about 5 minutes or until golden brown.

4. Serve warm.

Nutrition: **Calories:** 249; **Protein:** 12g

Carbs: 30g; **Fat:** 10g; **Sodium:** (Na) 32mg

Potassium: (K) 398mg; **Phosphorus:** 190mg

197. SAVORY BAGEL SEASONING CHAFFLES

♥ **Servings:** 2

Preparation Time: 10 Minutes

⏰ **Cooking Time:** 5 Minutes

Ingredients:

- ✓ 2 tablespoons Everything bagel seasoning
- ✓ 2 eggs
- ✓ 1 cup mozzarella cheese
- ✓ 1/2 cup grated parmesan

Directions:

1. Preheat the square waffle maker and grease it with cooking spray.

2. Mix together the eggs, mozzarella cheese, and grated cheese in a bowl.

3. Pour half of the batter into the waffle maker.

4. Sprinkle one tablespoon of the everything bagel seasoning over the batter.

5. Close the lid.

6. Cook the chaffles for about 3-4 minutes.

7. Repeat with the remaining batter.

8. Serve hot and enjoy!

Nutrition: **Calories:** 64; **Fat:** 3.1; **Fiber:** 3

Carbs: 7.1; **Protein:** 2.8

198. DRIED HERBS CHAFFLE

♥ **Servings:** 2

Preparation Time: 6 Minutes

⏰ **Cooking Time:** 8 Minutes

Ingredients:

- ✓ 1 organic egg, beaten
- ✓ ½ cup Cheddar cheese, shredded
- ✓ 1 tablespoon almond flour
- ✓ A pinch of dried thyme, crushed
- ✓ A pinch of dried rosemary, crushed

Directions:

1. Preheat a mini waffle maker and then grease it.

2. In a bowl, place all the ingredients and beat until well combined.

3. Place half of the mixture into the preheated waffle iron and cook for about four minutes or until golden brown.

4. Repeat with the remaining mixture.

5. Serve warm.

Nutrition: **Calories:** 80; **Fat:** 2.5; **Fiber:** 3.9

Carbs: 10.9; **Protein:** 4

199. ZUCCHINI & BASIL CHAFFLES

Servings: 2

Preparation Time: 6 Minutes

Cooking Time: 10 Minutes

Ingredients:

- ✓ 1 organic egg, beaten
- ✓ ¼ cup Mozzarella cheese, shredded
- ✓ 2 tablespoons Parmesan cheese, grated
- ✓ ½ of a small zucchini, grated and squeezed
- ✓ ¼ teaspoon dried basil, crushed
- ✓ Freshly ground black pepper, as required

Directions:

1. Preheat a mini waffle maker and then grease it.

2. In a medium bowl, place all ingredients and mix until well combined.

3. Place half of the mixture into the preheated waffle iron and cook for about 4-5 minutes or until golden brown.

4. Repeat with the remaining mixture.

5. Serve warm.

Nutrition: **Calories:** 43; **Fat:** 3.4; **Fiber:** 1.7 **Carbs:** 3.4; **Protein:** 1.3

200. HASH BROWN CHAFFLE

Servings: 2

Preparation Time: 6 Minutes

Cooking Time: 10 Minutes

Ingredients:

- ✓ 1 large jicama root, peeled and shredded
- ✓ ½ medium onion, minced
- ✓ 2 garlic cloves, pressed
- ✓ 1 cup cheddar shredded cheese
- ✓ 2 eggs
- ✓ Salt and pepper, to taste

Directions:

1. Place jicama in a colander, sprinkle with two teaspoons salt, and let drain.

2. Squeeze out all excess liquid.

3. Microwave jicama for 5-8 minutes.

4. Mix ¾ of cheese and all other ingredients in a bowl.

5. Sprinkle 1-2 teaspoon cheese on the waffle maker, add three tablespoons of the mixture, and top with 1-2 teaspoon cheese.

6. Cook for 5-minutes, or until done.

7. Remove and repeat for the remaining batter.

8. Serve while hot with your preferred toppings.

Nutrition: **Calories**: 81; **Fat**: 4.2; **Fiber**: 6.5

Carbs: 11.1; **Protein**: 1.9

Conclusion

The ketogenic diet is an incredibly great way to lose weight and get rid of the fat layers around your arms, legs, stomach, and even your internal organs. The results of the burned fat are visible within a couple of weeks (if you stick to the recommended foods and don't cheat).

Weight loss is one of the most popular reasons why people start this diet is because it is a sure way to lose weight and not face the yo-yo effect. It is because the keto diet offers a plethora of delicious foods and recipes that will keep you full and kill off your cravings for junk food and food rich in carbs or sugar.

Nutritionists and doctors often recommend it to overweight people who must lose weight, not for aesthetic reasons but because their life and health are in danger. This diet is great even if you don't want to lose weight. Just switch to keto meals, and you will lower the risk of many nasty diseases. Also, you will eat healthy and balanced food free of excessive amounts of sodium, sugar, carbs, and unhealthy oils and fats. As your body increases the ketone levels, all the stored fats will turn into energy. So, the gain is double—weight and fat loss, and a healthy and energized body.

The anti-inflammatory effect is true. No matter how crazy it sounds, once you start following the keto diet and the ketones in your body increase and fats are the primary energy source, you will release less reactive oxygen species and free radicals, which are dangerous for any human being. Free radicals and reactive oxygen species are the main reasons why today, people are more prone to deadly illnesses such as cancer. The less sugar you consume, the lower the risk is for you to develop inflammatory processes of any kind, to put it simply.

The diet helps decrease sugar levels in the blood. The more carbohydrates you eat, the more they are turned into blood sugar. You do not have to be a doctor to know that high blood sugar levels are the main reason why the insulin in the body rises. Increased insulin levels are the main reason for type 2 diabetes. Since this diet recommends foods that are deficient in carbohydrates, your body becomes supplied with a high level of fats, which have now become its primary energy source.

The fats you consume, and the fats that have already been stored are slowly burned and turned into energy for your brain. As the liver transforms the fats into ketones, there is a low level of insulin in the body. You are in control of insulin levels and prevent yourself from the risk of diabetes. If you have this condition, then you are controlling the insulin and prevent it from growing higher and damaging your health.

The diet helps to have better brain activity; there are far more benefits with the keto diet than weight loss, dropped levels of insulin in your body. You will feel more energized, but also low-carb food will put your brain in better shape. Now, if you are a young person, perhaps you don't think that this is necessary for you, but improved brain activity is super important for older people. No matter if you are a young or older person, the keto diet will improve your memory, and you will have an easier time learning and understanding new things. The great thing is that you will have an easier time keeping your thoughts in a better state, and your mood swings will significantly improve.

This is all thanks to the lower levels of insulin in your body. Studies have shown when you have lower insulin levels, you are practically slowing down the oxidative stress, and it decreases (which is in direct correlation with a person's aging process and lifespan).

Regarding Cancer, you read that the keto diet worked well for epileptic and diabetic patients, but such a diet is quite miraculous for cancer patients and survivors too. Cancer patients must be more careful with their food, so their doctors usually recommend a healthier diet. Keto is not a new thing for treating cancer patients or survivors.

Cancer cells grow faster when the body is provided with lots of sugar and carbs that will be turned into glucose. The Keto diet restricts such foods; therefore, the cancer cells are no longer fed with foods that cause even bigger damage. Also, it is highly important to eat food rich in fat because fat provides better energy than carbs, which for cancer patients is crucial. They need to regain their energy and strength, especially after chemotherapy.

The diet increases immunity; if you have immunity issues, the best way to boost it is to switch to foods that will reduce the risk for you to catch common colds, flu, and other inflammations. Everybody needs a strong immune system. If this diet showed a gradual improvement of the immune system in cancer patients only after one month, you could only imagine how well a healthy person will react to keto foods.

It increases a good mental state. Autistic and bipolar patients are often advised to eat keto meals. Many studies show that treating autistic children with the Ketogenic diet for six months showed improvement in their mental and behavioral state. Keeping patients with autism or any other mental disorder in a good mental state needs is crucial. The keto diet is a perfect way to keep you in a stable mood and will not cause you mood swings (which unfortunately often happens when you eat food rich in carbs).

Talking about Epilepsy, the Ketogenic diet was primarily developed to treat epileptic children with frequent seizures. About one century ago, when keto was first discovered, it significantly reduced epileptic seizures in children, ever since it is recommended for patients with epilepsy.

It is good for your general health. Your diet can either kill you or cure you. It does not matter why you start following the keto diet (weight loss, immunity system, energy, strength, etc.); it will improve your general health for the better. The keto meals are delicious enough, so that can be a good reason to start following it even if you don't need to lose weight. You will let go of your old eating habits, become more aware of what you eat, and your energy levels will rise.

The keto diet will provide you with the most important nutrients, healthy fats, proteins, and fiber, healthy oils (coconut, avocado, and olive).

You will see that there are many healthy and great food substitutes for all the unhealthy and junk food you used to eat. As the ketones in your body rise, your immune system will be put in balance, your skin, hair, and nails will become stronger, and you will keep your cholesterol and triglycerides under control.

Finally, one of the biggest reasons to start following this diet is the fact that there are no side effects; keto meals cannot harm you at all. The biggest challenge will last for a few days when you will quit eating carbohydrates (bread, pasta, sweets), but once you get used to the new foods, you will not even think twice about going back.

Made in the USA
Thornton, CO
09/09/24 19:43:45

1a719ab1-99ba-42c0-b7fd-5ee74e35210bR03